Place 2⅛ × 2⅛ **Sticky Notes** here
for a convenient and refillable note

✓ HIPAA Compliant
✓ OSHA Compliant

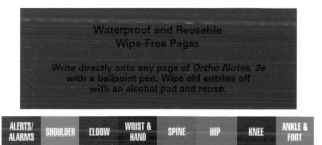

Waterproof and Reusable
Wipe-Free Pages

Write directly onto any page of *Ortho Notes, 2e*
with a ballpoint pen. Wipe old entries off
with an alcohol pad and reuse.

| ALERTS/ALARMS | SHOULDER | ELBOW | WRIST & HAND | SPINE | HIP | KNEE | ANKLE & FOOT |

Look for our other Davis's Notes Titles

For a complete list of Davis's Notes and
other titles for health care providers, visit www.fadavis.com

2nd Edition

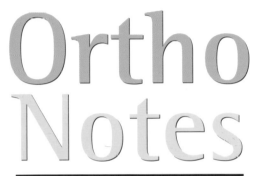

Ortho Notes

Clinical Examination Pocket Guide

Dawn Gulick, PhD, PT, ATC, CSCS

Purchase additional copies of this book at your health science bookstore or directly from F.A. Davis by shopping online at www.fadavis.com or by calling 800-323-3555 (US) or 800-665-1148 (CAN)

A Davis Note's Book

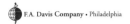
F.A. Davis Company • Philadelphia

F. A. Davis Company
1915 Arch Street
Philadelphia, PA 19103
www.fadavis.com

Printed in China

Last digit indicates print number: 10 9 8 7 6 5 4 3 2

Publisher: Margaret Biblis

Acquisitions Editor: Melissa Duffield
Manager of Content Development: George W. Lang
Developmental Editor: Yvonne Gillam
Art and Design Manager: Carolyn O'Brien

As new scientific information becomes available through basic and clinical research, recom-
mended treatments and drug therapies undergo changes. The author(s) and publisher have done
everything possible to make this book accurate, up to date, and in accord with accepted standards at the time of publication. The author(s), editors, and publisher are not responsible for
errors or omissions or for consequences from application of the book, and make no warranty,
expressed or implied, in regard to the contents of the book. Any practice described in this book
should be applied by the reader in accordance with professional standards of care used in regard
to the unique circumstances that may apply in each situation. The reader is advised always to
check product information (package inserts) for changes and new information regarding dose
and contraindications before administering any drug. Caution is especially urged when using
new or infrequently ordered drugs.

Authorization to photocopy items for internal or personal use, or the internal or personal use of
specific clients, is granted by F. A. Davis Company for users registered with the Copyright
Clearance Center (CCC) Transactional Reporting Service, provided that the fee of $.25 per copy is
paid directly to CCC, 222 Rosewood Drive, Danvers, MA 01923. For those organizations that have
been granted a photocopy license by CCC, a separate system of payment has been arranged. The
fee code for users of the Transactional Reporting Service is: 8036-2067-5/09 0 + $.25.

Medical Screening

Have you ever experienced or been told you have any of the following conditions?

Cancer	Chronic bronchitis
Diabetes	Pneumonia
High blood pressure	Emphysema
Fainting or dizziness	Migraine headaches
Chest pain	Anemia
Shortness of breath	Stomach ulcers
Blood clot	AIDS/HIV
Stroke	Hemophilia
Kidney disease	Guillain-Barré syndrome
Urinary tract infection	Gout
Allergies (latex, food, drug)	Thyroid problems
Asthma	Multiple sclerosis
Osteoporosis	Tuberculosis
Rheumatic/scarlet fever	Fibromyalgia
Hepatitis/jaundice	Pregnancy
Polio	Hernia
Head injury/concussion	Depression
Epilepsy or seizures	Frequent falls
Parkinson's disease	Bowel/bladder problems
Arthritis	

Have you ever had any of the following procedures?

X-ray	Blood test(s)
CT scan	Biopsy
MRI	EMG or NCV
Bone scan	EKG or stress test
Urine analysis	Surgery

Normal Vital Signs & Pathologies That Influence Them

Age	Infant	Child	Adolescent	Adult & Elderly	Increases Due to:	Decreases Due to:
T	98.2°	98.6°	98.6°	98.6°	Infection, exercise, ↑ blood sugar	↓ Hematocrit & hemoglobin, narcotics, ↓ blood sugar, aging
HR	80–180	75–140	50–100	60–100	Infection, ↓ Hematocrit & hemoglobin, ↓ blood sugar, anxiety, anemia, pain, ↓ K⁺, exercise	Narcotics, acute MI, ↑ K⁺
RR	30–50	20–40	15–22	10–20	Infection, ↓ Hematocrit & hemoglobin, ↑ blood sugar, anxiety, pain, acute MI, asthma, exercise	Narcotics
SBP	73	90	115	<130	↑ blood sugar, CAD, anxiety, pain, exercise (SBP only)	↓ Hematocrit & hemoglobin, ↓ K, narcotics, acute MI, anemia
DBP	55	57	70	<85		

Signs/Symptoms of Emergency Situations

- SBP ≥180 mm Hg or ≤90 mm Hg
- DBP ≥110 mm Hg
- Resting HR >100 bpm
- Resting RR >30 bpm
- Sudden change in mentation
- Facial pain with intractable headache
- Sudden onset of angina or arrhythmia
- Abdominal rebound tenderness
- Black, tarry, or bloody stools

Generalized Systemic Red Flags

- Insidious onset with no known mechanism of injury
- Symptoms out of proportion to injury
- No change in symptoms despite positioning or rest
- Symptoms persist beyond expected healing time
- Recent or current fever, chills, night sweats, infection
- Unexplained weight loss, pallor, nausea, B&B changes (constitutional symptoms)
- Headache or visual changes
- Bilateral symptoms
- Pigmentation changes, edema, rash, nail changes, weakness, numbness, tingling, burning
- Psoas test for pelvic pathology = supine, SLR to 30° & resist hip flexion; (+) test for pelvic inflammation or infection is lower quadrant abdominal pain, hip or back pain is a ( ) test
- Blumberg's sign = rebound tenderness for visceral pathology—in supine select a site away from the painful area & place your hand perpendicular & push down deep & slow then lift up quickly; (–) = no pain; (+) = pain on release
- (+) McBurney's point (appendix) = ⅓–½ the distance between the Ⓡ ASIS & umbilicus
- (+) Kehr's sign (spleen) = violent Ⓛ shoulder pain

Visceral Innervation & Referral Patterns

Segmental Innervation	Viscera	Referral Pattern(s)
C3–5	Diaphragm	C-spine
T1–5	Heart	Anterior neck, chest, left UE
T4–6	Esophagus	Substernal & upper abdominal
T5–6	Lungs	T-spine
T6–10	Stomach	Upper abdomen & T-spine
	Pancreas	Upper abdomen, low T-spine, & upper L-spine
	Bile duct	Upper abdomen, mid T-spine
T7–9	Gallbladder	Right UQ, right T-spine
	Liver	Right T-spine
T7–10	Small intestine	Mid T-spine
T10–11	Testes/Ovaries	Lower abdomen & sacrum
T10–L1	Kidney	L-spine, abdomen
T10–L1 S2–4	Uterus Prostate	T/L & L/S junction Sacrum, testes, T/L jctn
T11–L2, S2–4	Ureter	Groin, suprapubic, medial thigh
	Bladder	Sacral apex, suprapubic

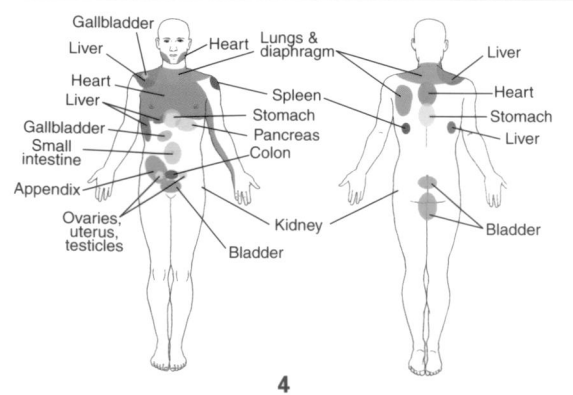

4

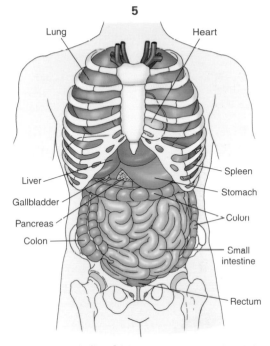

Lung

Heart

Liver

Spleen

Gallbladder

Stomach

Pancreas

Colon

Colon

Small intestine

Rectum

Source: From Gulick, D. Screening Notes: Rehabilitation Specialist's Pocket Guide. FA Davis, Philadelphia, 2006, pages 11-12.

Early Warning Signs of Cancer

"CAUTIONS" = Red Flags of Cancer

C = Change in bowel & bladder lasting longer than 7–10 days
A = A sore that fails to heal in 6 weeks
U = Unusual bleeding or discharge
T = Thickening/lump (breast or elsewhere)
I = Indigestion, difficulty swallowing, early satiety
O = Obvious change in wart or mole
- **A** = Asymmetrical shape
- **B** = Border irregularities
- **C** = Color—pigmentation is not uniform
- **D** = Diameter >6 mm (bigger than a pencil eraser)
- **E** = Evolution (change in status)
N = Nagging cough or hoarseness (rust-colored sputum)
S = Supplemental signs/symptoms
- 10–15 lb wt loss in 10–14 days
- Changes in vital signs
- Frequent infections (respiratory or urinary)
- + change in DTRs
- + proximal muscle weakness
- + night pain
- + pathologic fracture
- >45 years old

Cardiovascular Signs to Discontinue Exercise

- Resting HR <40 or >130
- Irregular pulse; palpitations
- > 6 arrhythmias per hour
- Blood glucose >250 mg/dL
- O_2 saturation <90%
- Temp >100°F
- SBP >250 or DBP >120 mm Hg
- Fall in SBP >10 mm Hg
- Cognitive changes
- Cold, clammy, cyanotic
- PO_2 <60; hemoglobin <8 g/dL
- Dyspnea; orthopnea
- Dizziness, syncope
- Bilateral leg or foot edema
- Chest pain (with or without UE radiation)
- Isolated ® biceps or mid-thoracic pain in females

Signs & Symptoms of Specific Organ Pathology

Pulmonary

- Cough with or without blood
- Sputum
- SOB or DOE
- Clubbing of nails
- Chest pain
- Wheezing
- Pain with deep inspiration
- Pain ↑ when recumbent & ↓ on involved side
- ↓ O_2 saturation
- Signs of a PE
  - Pleural pain
  - SOB
  - Rapid RR
  - Rapid HR
  - Coughing up blood

Hepatic

- ⓇUQ pain
- Weight loss
- Ascites/LE edema
- Carpal tunnel syndrome (bilateral)
- Intermittent pruritus
- Weakness & fatigue
- Dark urine/clay-colored stools
- Asterixis (liver flap) = flapping tremor resulting from the inability to maintain wrist extension with forearm supported
- Jaundice, bruising, yellow sclera of the eye
- Pain referral to T-spine between scapula, Ⓡ shoulder, Ⓡ upper trap, Ⓡ subscapular region

Gastrointestinal

- Epigastric pain with radiation to the back
- Blood or dark, tarry stool
- Fecal incontinence or urgency
- Tenderness @ McBurney's point
- Pain/symptoms that change with eating
- Nausea, vomiting, bloating
- Diarrhea or absence of bowel mov't
- Food may help or aggravate px
- Weight loss, loss of appetite

Renal

- (+) Murphy's test = percussion over kidney
- Fever; chills
- Blood in urine (hematuria)
- Cloudy or foul-smelling urine
- Painful or frequent urination
- Pain is constant (stones)
- Back pain at the level of the kidneys
- Costovertebral angle tenderness

Prostate

- Men >50 yo
- Difficulty starting or stopping urine flow
- Change in frequency
- Nocturia
- Incontinence/dribbling
- PSA level >4 ng/mL
- Sexual dysfunction

Gynecological

- Cyclic pain
- Abnormal blooding
- Nausea, vomiting
- Vaginal discharge
- Chronic constipation
- Low BP (blood loss)
- Missed or irregular periods

Tasks That May Aggravate & Incriminate Visceral Pathology

- GB = forward bending
- Kidney = lean to affected side
- Pancreas = sit up or lean forward
- Esophagus = swallowing
- GI = eating
- Heart = cold air or exertion
- Renal = side bending away from involved side

Signs & Symptoms of Hyperglycemia

- Blood glucose >180 mg/dL
- Skin is dry & flushed
- Fruity breath odor
- Blurred vision
- Dizziness
- Weakness
- Nausea
- Vomiting
- Cramping
- Increased urination
- LOC/seizure

Signs & Symptoms of Hypoglycemia

- Blood glucose <50–60 mg/dL
- Skin is pale, cool, diaphoretic
- Disoriented or agitated
- Headache
- Slurred speech
- Tachycardic
- LOC

Asthmatic Response(s)

- Coughing, wheezing
- Substernal chest tightness
- Use of accessory muscles of respiration
- RR >24 bpm
- Peak flow <80% predicted or baseline value
- After an asthma attack, FEV1 peak flow should ↑ by >15% within 5 min of use of inhaler

Signs & Symptoms of Marfan's Syndrome (inherited autosomal dominant disorder)

- Disproportionately long arms, legs, fingers, & toes (tall—lower body longer than upper body)
- Long skull with frontal prominence
- Kyphoscoliosis
- Pectus chest (concave)
- Slender ↓ sub-q fat
- Weak tendons, ligaments, & joint capsules with joint hypermobility
- Defective heart valves = murmur
- High incidence of dissecting aortic aneurysm
- Hernia
- Sleep apnea
- Dislocation of eye lens; myopia
- "Thumb sign" = oppose the thumb across the palm, if tip of thumb extends beyond the palm, the test is (+)

Signs & Symptoms of Depression

- Sadness; frequent/unexplained crying
- Feelings of guilt, helplessness, or hopelessness
- Suicide ideations
- Problems sleeping
- Fatigue or decreased energy; apathy
- Loss of appetite; weight loss/gain
- Difficulty concentrating, remembering, & making decisions

Signs & Symptoms of Lyme's Disease

Note: This is a multisystemic inflammatory condition. The transmission of the tick spirochete takes ~ 48 hrs. Blood work is used to confirm the disease, not to diagnose it. Clinician should r/o GBS, MS, & FMS.

Early Localized Stage
- Rash with onset of erythema within 7–14 days (range is 3–30 days)
- Rash may be solid red expanding rash or a central spot with rings (Bull's-eye)
- Average diameter of rash is 5"–6"
- Rash may or may not be warm to palpation
- Rash is usually not painful or itchy
- Fever
- Malaise
- Headache
- Muscle aches
- Joint pain

Early Disseminated Stage
- ≥ 2 rashes not @ the bite site
- Migrating pain
- Headache
- Stiff neck
- Facial palsy
- Numbness/tingling into extremities
- Abnormal pulse
- Sore throat
- Visual changes

- 100°–102° fever
- Severe fatigue

Late Stage

- Arthritis of 1–2 larger joints
- Neurological changes—disorientation, confusion, dizziness, mental "fog," numbness in extremities
- Visual impairment
- Cardiac irregularities

Dementia Scales

Score	Maximum	Task
	5 5	**Orientation:** What is the (year) (season) (date) (day) (month)? Where are we (state) (country) (town) (building) (floor)?
	3	**Registration:** Name 3 objects: 1 second to say each. Ask the patient all 3 after you have said them. Give 1 pt for each correct answer. Repeat them until he/she learns all 3. Count & record trials: _____
	5	**Attention & Calculation:** Serial 7s. Score 1 point for each correct answer. Stop after 5 answers. (Alternative question: Spell "world" backward.)
	3	**Recall:** Ask for the 3 objects repeated above. Give 1 point for each correct answer.
	2 1 3 1 1 1	**Language:** Name a pencil & watch. Repeat the following, "No, ifs, ands, or buts." Follow a 3-stage command: "Take a paper in your hand, fold it in half, & put it on the floor." Read & obey the following: "Close your eyes." Write a sentence. Copy the design shown:
	30	**Total score (Normal ≥24)**

Deep Tendon Reflexes

Grade	Response	Jendrassik's Maneuver
0	Absent; areflexia	For UE = patient crosses LEs at ankles & then isometrically abducts LEs
1+	Decreased; hyporeflexia	
2+	Normal	For LE = patient interlocks fingertips & then isometrically pulls elbows apart
3+	Hyperactive; brisk	
4+	Hyperactive with clonus	

Cranial Nerves

Nerve	Function	Test
I. Olfactory	Smell	Identify odors with eyes closed
II. Optic	Vision	Test peripheral vision with 1 eye covered
III. Oculomotor	Eye movement & pupillary reaction	Peripheral vision, eye chart, reaction to light
IV. Trochlear	Eye movement	Test ability to depress & adduct eye
V. Trigeminal	Face sensation & mastication	Face sensation & clench teeth
VI. Abducens	Eye movement	Test ability to abduct eye past midline
VII. Facial	Facial muscles & taste	Close eyes & smile; detect various tastes—sweet, sour, salty, bitter
VIII. Vestibulocochlear (Acoustic)	Hearing & balance	Hearing, feet together, eyes open/closed x 5 sec; test for past-pointing
IX. Glossopharyngeal	Swallow, voice, gag reflex	Swallow & say "ahh" Use tongue depressor to elicit gag reflex
X. Vagus	Swallow, voice, gag reflex	
XI. Spinal Accessory	SCM & trapezius	Rotate/SB neck; shrug shoulders
XII. Hypoglossal	Tongue mov't	Protrude tongue (watch for lateral deviation)

Neural Tissue Provocation Tests (NTPT)

MEDIAN NERVE TEST

Position: Supine or sitting with contralateral cervical SB & ipsilateral shoulder depressed

Technique: Extend UE in plane of scapula with elbow extended, forearm supinated, & wrist/fingers extended

Interpretation: + test = pain or paresthesia into median nerve distribution of UE

Statistics: Sensitivity = 94%; specificity = 22%

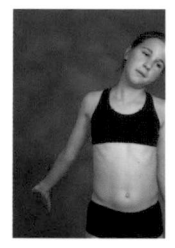

RADIAL NERVE TEST

Position: Supine or sitting with contralateral cervical SB & ipsilateral shoulder depressed

Technique: Extend UE with elbow extended, forearm pronated, wrist flexed, & fingers extended

Interpretation: + test = pain or paresthesia into radial nerve distribution of UE

Statistics: Sensitivity = 97%; specificity = 33%

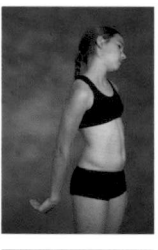

ULNAR NERVE TEST

Position: Supine or sitting with ipsilateral shoulder depressed

Technique: Abduct shoulder to 90° with ER, flex elbow, pronate forearm, extend wrist/fingers in an attempt to place the palm of the hand on the ipsilateral ear

Interpretation: + test = pain or paresthesia into ulnar nerve distribution of UE

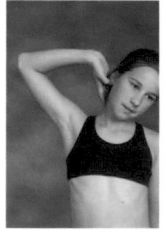

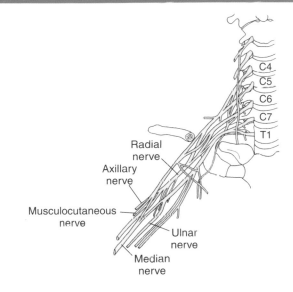

Radial
nerve

Axillary
nerve

Musculocutaneous
nerve

Ulnar
nerve

Median
nerve

C4
C5
C6
C7
T1

Axillary Nerve

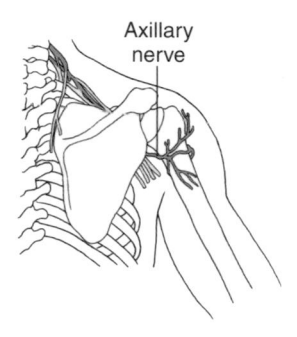

Axillary nerve

Musculocutaneous Nerve

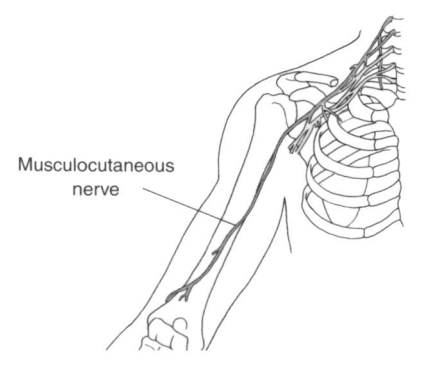

Musculocutaneous nerve

Radial Nerve

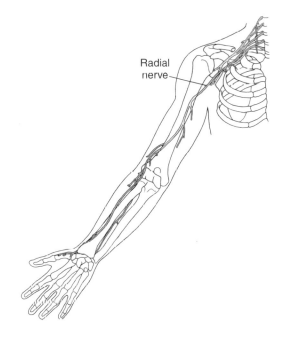

Radial
nerve

Median Nerve

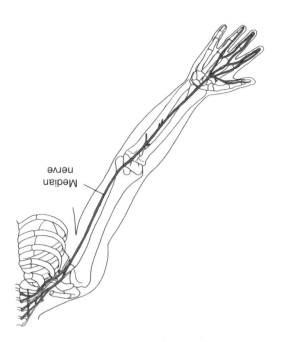

Median
nerve

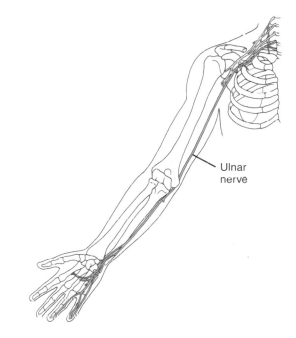

Ulnar
nerve

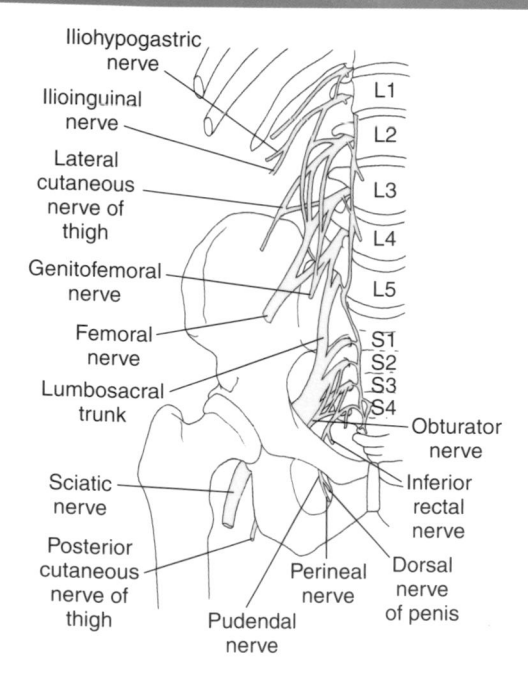

Iliohypogastric nerve

Ilioinguinal nerve

Lateral cutaneous nerve of thigh

Genitofemoral nerve

Femoral nerve

Lumbosacral trunk

Sciatic nerve

Posterior cutaneous nerve of thigh

Pudendal nerve

Perineal nerve

Dorsal nerve of penis

Inferior rectal nerve

Obturator nerve

L1
L2
L3
L4
L5
S1
S2
S3
S4

Femoral, Obturator, Sciatic, Tibial, & Common Peroneal Nerve

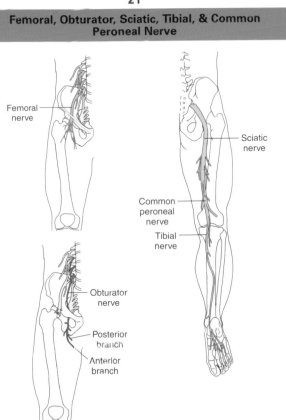

Femoral nerve

Sciatic nerve

Common peroneal nerve

Tibial nerve

Obturator nerve

Posterior branch

Anterior branch

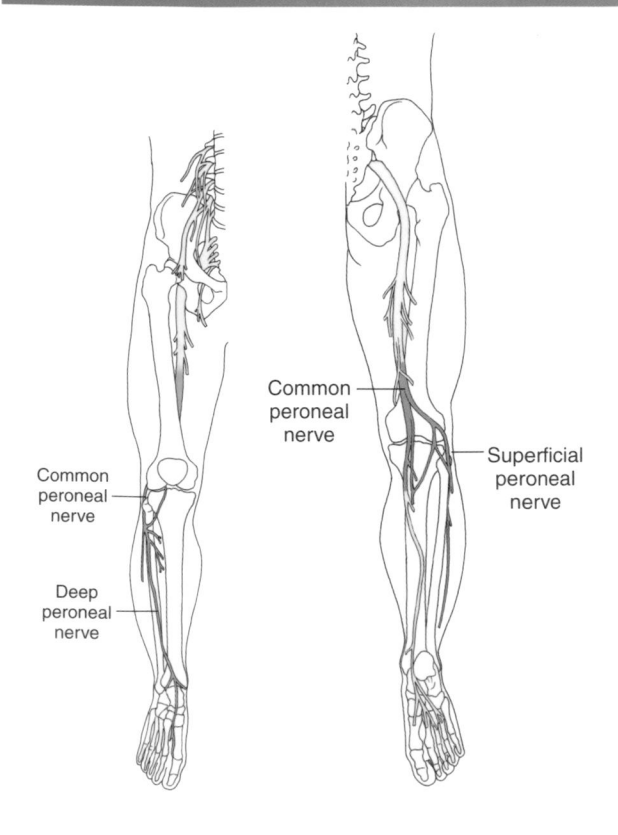

Common peroneal nerve

Deep peroneal nerve

Common peroneal nerve

Superficial peroneal nerve

Pharmacologic Summary by Drug Classification

Nonnarcotic Analgesic

Indications = Pain, fever

Generic name (Brand names)	Adverse reactions (Most frequent are **bolded**)	Interactions
Acetaminophen • Tylenol • Anacin-3 • Liquiprin • Panadol • Acephen • Tempra	**Upset stomach, rash, bruising, anemia** Doses >15g are toxic to liver & kidney; may be fatal	Barbiturates = ↓ effects & ↑ liver toxicity Warfarin = ↑ anticoagulant effect Caffeine = ↑ analgesic effects Alcohol = ↑ risk of liver damage (not recommended if consuming ≥ 3 glasses of alcohol/day

Analgesic & NSAID

Indications = RA, OA, JRA, pain, fever, prevent thrombosis, reduce risk of MI, TIA, CVA
Anti-inflammatory doses are > analgesic doses

Generic name (Brand names)	Adverse reactions (Most frequent are bolded)	Interactions
Acetylsalicylic acid (ASA) • Aspirin • Ecotrin • Empirin • Bayer • Aspergum	**Not recommended for children** **Tinnitus, nausea, prolonged** **bleeding time, rash,** GI distress, bruising	**All NSAIDs:** • Can ↓ cardioprotective effects of low-dose aspirin • Can ↑ risk of bleeding when used with ginkgo, vitamin E, warfarin, Plavix, & heparin • Can ↑ BP (COX-2 inhibitors ↑ BP to a lesser extent than nonselectives) • Can ↑ neurotoxicity when used with lithium
Ibuprofen • Motrin • Nuprin • Advil	GI px, dyspepsia, nausea, dizziness, rash, hepatitis, h/a	
Sulindac • Clinoril	**Not recommended for children** **GI px,** h/a, rash, constipation, dizziness, liver damage, epider- mal necrosis syndrome	• Can produce acute renal failure • Are gastric irritants & can produce nephrotoxicity
Meloxicam (preferential inhibition of COX-2 over COX-1)	Seizures, cardiac arrhythmias, MI, hemorrhage, asthma, erythema, anaphylactic reaction, anxiety, abdominal pain, coughing	

Exercise concerns: Negative effect on myogenesis & regeneration (anabolic effects)

Analgesic & NSAID—cont'd

Indications = RA, OA, JRA, pain, fever, prevent thrombosis, reduce risk of MI, TIA, CVA
Anti-inflammatory doses are > analgesic doses

Generic name (Brand names)	Adverse reactions (Most frequent are bolded)	Interactions
Naproxen	**Not recommended for children**	**All NSAIDs:**
• Naprosyn	**Tinnitus,** GI px, constipation, h/a, dizziness,	• Can ↓ cardioprotective effects of low-dose aspirin
• Anaprox	rash, edema, ecchymoses	• Can ↑ risk of bleeding when used with ginkgo, vitamin E, warfarin, Plavix, & heparin
Diflunisal	**Not recommended for children**	• Can ↑ BP (COX-2 inhibitors ↑ BP to a lesser extent than nonselectives)
• Dolobid	GI px, diarrhea, dyspepsia, rash, h/a, dizziness, insomnia	• Can ↑ neurotoxicity when used with lithium
Piroxicam	**Not recommended for children**	• Can produce acute renal failure
• Feldene	**Greater risk of GI bleeding than other NSAIDs** Dizziness, h/a, edema, rash, pruritus, hepatitis	• Are gastric irritants & can produce nephrotoxicity

Exercise concerns: Negative effect on myogenesis & regeneration (anabolic effects)

Continued

Analgesic & NSAID—cont'd

Indications = RA, OA, JRA, pain, fever, prevent thrombosis, reduce risk of MI, TIA, CVA
Anti-inflammatory doses are > analgesic doses

Generic name (Brand names)	Adverse reactions (Most frequent are bolded)	Interactions
Indomethacin • Indocin	**H/a**, drowsy, dizziness, nausea, GI px, constipation, pancreatitis	**All NSAIDs:** • Can ↓ cardioprotective effects of low-dose aspirin
Etodolac • Lodine	Not recommended for children **Dyspepsia**, slightly less GI px than other NSAID, nausea, diarrhea, CHF, dizziness, ↑ BP, blurred vision	• Can ↑ risk of bleeding when used with ginkgo, vitamin E, warfarin, Plavix, & heparin • Can ↑ BP (COX-2 inhibitors ↑ BP to a lesser extent than nonselectives)
Ketoprofen • Orudis	Not recommended for children **Dyspepsia**, h/a, dizziness, insomnia, tinnitus, peripheral edema	• Can ↑ neurotoxicity when used with lithium • Can produce acute renal failure • Are gastric irritants & can produce nephrotoxicity

Exercise concerns: Negative effect on myogenesis & regeneration (anabolic effects)

Analgesic & NSAID—cont'd

Indications = RA, OA, JRA, pain, fever, prevent thrombosis, reduce risk of MI, TIA, CVA
Anti-inflammatory doses are > analgesic doses

Generic name (Brand names)	Adverse reactions (Most frequent are **bolded**)	Interactions
Diclofenac • Voltaren • Cataflam	**Not recommended for children** **Nephrotic px**, GI px, h/a, edema, dizziness, hypoglycemia	**All NSAIDs:** • Can ↓ cardioprotective effects of low-dose aspirin • Can ↑ risk of bleeding when used with ginkgo, vitamin E, warfarin, Plavix, & heparin • Can ↑ BP (COX-2 inhibitors ↑ BP to a lesser extent than nonselectives) • Can ↑ neuro toxicity when used with lithium • Are gastric irritants & can produce nephrotoxicity
Nabumetone • Relafen	**Not recommended for children** **Abdominal pain, diarrhea, dyspepsia,** dizziness, h/a, dyspnea, diaphoresis	
Celecoxib (COX-2 inhib) • Celebrex	**Not recommended for children** h/a, GI px, dizziness, ↑ BP, erythema	

Exercise concerns: Negative effect on myogenesis & regeneration (anabolic effects), i.e., may delay muscle healing

*Narcotic Analgesic: APAP = Acetaminophen

Indication = Pain

Generic name (Brand names)	Adverse reactions (Most frequent are **bolded**)	Interactions
APAP/hydrocodone** • Vicodin • Lortab	**Dizziness, nausea,** vomiting, confusion, constipation, rash, pruritus, depression	Antihistamines, antipsychotics, or antianxiety agents = ↑ CNS depression MAO inhibitors= ↑ effects
APAP/codeine** • Tylenol #3	**Nausea,** drowsiness, constipation, nausea, vomiting, SOB, pruritus ↓ respiration (body builds up tolerance after 2 wks)	Antipsychotics, antianxiety agents, or alcohol = ↑ CNS depression Anticholinergics with codeine = paralytic ileus
APAP/oxycodone • Percocet • Tylox	**Lightheaded, dizziness, nausea, vomiting, apnea, respiratory distress, hypotension,** rash, constipation, pruritus	Muscle relaxers = ↑ CNS effects

Exercise concerns: Reduced exercise capacity due to respiratory depression especially with COPD; guard ambulation to prevent falls

*ALL opioids are addicting; withdrawal symptoms may appear in 6–10 hours & last 5 days. Symptoms may include body aches, diarrhea, fever, gooseflesh, insomnia, irritability, loss of appetite, nausea, vomiting, runny nose, shivering, & stomach cramps.
**Should not be taken w th MAO inhibitors.

*Narcotic Analgesic: ASA = Aspirin

Indication = Pain

Generic name (Brand names)	Adverse reactions (Most frequent are **bolded**)	Interactions (All interaction effects of ASA apply)
ASA/codeine* • Empirin with codeine **Take with food**	**Dizziness, nausea, ↓ respiration, constipation, tinnitus,** h/a, vomiting, pruritus, rash	MAO inhibitors, insulin, anticoagulants, methotrexate, or sulfonamides = ↑ effects NSAIDs = peptic ulcers Alcohol = ↑ CNS depression
ASA/oxycodore • Percodan	**Lightheaded, nausea, dizziness,** vomiting, euphoria, pruritus, apnea, constipation, circulatory depression, hemorrhage, hypotension	Muscle relaxant = ↑ CNS effects, impair judgment Analgesics, phenothiazines, tranquilizers, or alcohol = ↑ CNS depression ACE inhibitors = ↓ pain relief Anticoagulant or NSAID = ↑ bleeding Methotrexate = ↑ toxicity

Exercise concerns: Negative effects on myogenesis & regeneration (anabolic effects)

*ALL opioids are addicting; withdrawal symptoms may appear in 6-10 hours & last 5 days. Symptoms may include body aches, diarrhea, fever, gooseflesh, insomnia, irritability, loss of appetite, nausea, vomiting, runny nose, shivering, & stomach cramps.
**Should not be taken with MAO inhibitors.

Muscle Relaxers/Antispasmodics

Indications = Manage spasticity (muscle tone), reduce muscle guarding

Generic name (Brand names)	Adverse reactions (Most frequent are **bolded**)	Interactions
Baclofen • Lioresal	**Drowsiness, nausea, dizziness, weakness, confusion,** vomiting, high fever, h/a, rash, paresthesias	CNS depressants or alcohol = ↑ depression
Carisoprodol • Soma (addictive)	**Orthostatic hypotension, drowsiness, dizziness,** h/a, vertigo, agitation, insomnia	CNS depressants or alcohol = ↑ depression
Cyclobenzaprine • Flexeril (use not recommended for > 2–3 wks)	**Drowsiness, dry mouth, dizziness,** arrhythmias, confusion, transient visual hallucinations	CNS depressants or alcohol = ↑ depression MAO inhibitors or Tramadol = may cause seizures & death
Diazepam • Valium (long-term dependency)	**Drowsiness, pain, phlebitis at injection site,** dysarthria, constipation, ↓ HR, ↓ RR	CNS depressants or alcohol = ↑ depression Digoxin = risk of toxicity Smoking = may ↓ effects
Tizanidine • Zanaflex	**Somnolence, sedation, hypotension, dry mouth, UTI,** dizziness, bradycardia, constipation	Antihypertensives = ↓ BP Baclofen, alcohol, or other CNS depressant = additive effect Oral contraceptive = ↓ tizanidine clearance

Exercise concerns: Interferes with strengthening goals

ACE Inhibitors

Indication = High BP

Generic name (Brand names)	Adverse reactions (Most frequent are **bolded**)	Interactions
Captopril • Capoten	**Dry cough, rash**, dizziness, abdominal pain, neutropenia	Antacids = ↑ effects Digoxin = ↑ digoxin levels
Enalapril • Vasotec	**Weakness, dry cough**, dizziness, h/a, hypotension	Diuretics or phenothiazines = hypotension NSAIDs = ↓ antihypertensive effects
Lisinopril • Zestril • Prinivil	**Dizziness, nasal congestion, dry cough, orthostatic hypotension, diarrhea**, h/a, fatigue, nausea	Insulin = ↑ hypoglycemia Lithium = lithium toxicity
Fosinopril • Monopril	**Dizziness, dry cough**, h/a, fatigue, diarrhea, nausea	
Quinapril • Accupril	Somnolence, pruritus, dizziness, dry cough, hemorrhage	

Exercise concerns: No effect on exercise capacity

ACE Receptor Blockers

Indication = High BP

Generic name (Brand names)	Adverse reactions (Most frequent are **bolded**)	Interactions
Losartan K+ • Cozaar	**Dizziness, h/a, weakness, fatigue, chest pain, diarrhea, anemia, flu-like symptoms**	Due to ↑ K+ levels, should not be taken with K+ supplements, salt substitutes containing K+, or K+-sparing diuretics NSAIDs & ASA = ↓ antihypertensive effects
Candesartan • Atacand	**Dizziness, h/a, runny nose, URI**	
Irbesartan • Avapro	**Anxiety, chest pain, diarrhea, dizziness, flu, h/a, fatigue, nausea, upset stomach, sore throat, UTI, vomiting**	

Exercise concerns: No effect on exercise capacity

Ca++ Channel Blockers

Indication = Angina

Generic name (Brand names)	Adverse reactions (Most frequent are **bolded**)	Interactions
Diltiazem • Cardizem • Dilacor • Diltiaz	**LE edema, h/a, 1° heart block**, arrhythmia, bradycardia, nausea, rash, dizziness, fatigue, 1° heart block	Digoxin = elevated digitalis levels Anesthetics = ↑ anesthetic effects & depression of cardiac contractility Cyclosporine = ↑ cyclosporine level
• Tiazac		Diazepam = ↑ CNS depression
Verapamil • Calan	**Hypotension, AV block, constipation**, dizziness, nausea, h/a, arrhythmia, dyspnea	Beta-blockers = heart failure Cardiac glycoside = ↑ digitalis levels Antihypertensives = hypotension Cyclosporine = ↑ levels Grapefruit juice = ↑ drug level St. John's wort = ↓ drug level Alcohol = ↑ alcohol level
Amlodipine • Norvasc • Amvaz	**Edema**, h/a, fatigue, nausea, flushing, rash, LE edema, dizziness	When combined with another antihypertensive = hypotension When combined with an alpha blocker = hypotension & reflex tachycardia
Nifedipine • Procardia	**Dizziness, h/a, weakness, flushing, peripheral edema, nausea**	Verapamil = ↓ effects Antifungals or erythromycin = ↑ effects Fentanyl = severe hypotension Cimetidine = ↑ plasma level of nifedipine Beta blockers = hypotension Ginkgo or grapefruit juice = ↑ effects St. John's wort = ↓ drug effect

Exercise concerns: Drugs may cause arthralgia/myalgia that may negatively influence exercise capacity

*Beta Blockers/Antihypertensives

Indications = Angina, arrhythmias, hypertension

Generic name (Brand names)	Adverse reactions (Most frequent are bolded)	Interactions
Propranolol • Inderal • InnoPran	↑ **LDL cholesterol, bradycardia, fatigue, lethargy, hypotension,** lightheaded, abdominal cramping, rash, Raynaud's, bronchospasm in asthmatics	Verapamil or diltiazem = hypotension Epinephrine = severe peripheral vasoconstriction Insulin = hypoglycemia Phenothiazines = ↑ adverse reactions NSAIDs = ↓ antihypertensive effect
Atenolol • Tenormin	↑ **LDL cholesterol, dizziness, fatigue, hypotension, bradycardia,** nausea, LE pain, rash, bronchospasms, orthostatic hypotension	Ca^{++} channel blockers or prazosin = ↑ hypotension Cardiac glycosides = severe bradycardia Insulin = may alter dosage NSAIDs = ↓ antihypertensive effects
Timolol • Blocadren	↑ **LDL cholesterol,** bronchospasms, fatigue, bradycardia, extremity pain, weakness, impotence	NSAIDs = ↓ antihypertensive effect
Metoprolol • Lopressor • Toprol	↑ **LDL cholesterol, fatigue, dizziness, depression, hypotension,** bradycardia, nausea, rash, bronchospasms	Cardiac glycosides = severe bradycardia MAO inhibitors, cimetidine, hydralazine, prazosin, or verapamil = additive effects; hypotension & bradycardia
Labetalol • Normodyne • Trandate	↑ **LDL cholesterol,** dizziness, nausea, fatigue, hypotension	Cimetidine = ↑ labetalol plasma levels Verapamil = additive effects NSAIDs = ↓ antihypertensive effect

*Should not be taken with MAO inhibitors

*Beta Blockers/Antihypertensives—cont'd

Indications = Angina, arrhythmias, hypertension

Generic name (Brand names)	Adverse reactions (Most frequent are **bolded**)	Interactions
Carvedilol • Co-reg	↑ **LDL cholesterol**, asthenia, dizziness, fatigue, hypotension, diarrhea, hyperglycemia, wt gain, URI *May produce bronchoconstriction in patients with asthmatic conditions	Cimetidine = ↑ carvedilol plasma levels MAO inhibitors = bradycardia & ↓ BP Ca^{++} channel blockers = conduction disturbances NSAIDs = ↓ antihypertensive effect

Exercise concerns: As a result of a blunting of HR, exercise to 20 bpm above resting HR; beta blockers mask symptoms of & delay recovery from hypoglycemia

Antilipemics

Indications = Reduce LDL, total cholesterol, & triglyceride levels

Generic name (Brand names)	Adverse reactions (Most frequent are **bolded**)	Interactions
Atorvastatin • Lipitor	Constipation, muscle pain, flatulence, ↑ liver transaminase, dyspepsia, rhabdomyolysis	Antacids = ↓ plasma level of atorvastatin Digoxin or erythromycin = ↑ plasma level of atorvastatin BCP = ↑ plasma level of BCP Erythromycin, niacin, or antifungals = ↑ risk of myopathy

Exercise concerns: Muscle weakness & cramping, myalgia

Diuretics

Indications = Edema, hypertension

Generic name (Brand names)	Adverse reactions (Most frequent are **bolded**)	Interactions
Furosemide (loop diuretic) • Lasix	Dehydration, muscle cramps, hypokalemia, hypocalcemia (osteoporosis), cardia arrhythmias	Antihypertensives or Ca^{++} channel blocker = ↑ risk of hypotension & arrhythmias Loop + thiazide diuretic = ↑ risk of hypotension
Thiazide • Esidrix • Hydrodiuril • Lozol • Zaroxolyn	**Dizziness,** muscle weakness, cramps, thirst, hyperglycemia, stomach discomfort	& arrhythmias Cardiac glycosides = ↑ risk of digoxin toxicity with K$^+$ loss NSAIDs = inhibit diuretic response Sun = photosensitivity
K$^+$ sparing • Aldactone • Dyrenium	**Dizziness,** weakness, fatigue, h/a, diarrhea, dry mouth, muscle cramps	

Exercise concerns: Diminished exercise performance; limited muscle endurance; volume depletion; ↑ risk of heat-related illness; muscle cramps 2° hypokalemia

Antidepressants

Indication = Depression, OCD, anxiety

Generic name (Brand names)	Adverse reactions (Most frequent are **bolded**)	Interactions
Amitriptyline • Elavil	**Orthostatic hypotension, tachycardia, dry mouth**, stroke, arrhythmia, lethargy, confusion, dry mouth, urinary retention, blurred vision, constipation	Contraceptives = ↑ antidepressant level & ↑ tricyclic-induced akathisia Clonidine or epinephrine = extreme hypertension MAO inhibitors = severe excitation Quinolones = life-threatening arrhythmias (↑ QTc interval) Alcohol = CNS depression Sun = photosensitivity
Doxepin • Sinequan • Adapin • Zonalon	**Drowsiness, dizziness, dry mouth, orthostatic hypotension, blurred vision, tachycardia, diaphoresis, constipation, seizures**, confusion, urinary retention	Contraceptives = ↑ antidepressant level Clonidine or epinephrine = extreme hypertension MAO inhibitors = severe excitation Quinolones = life-threatening arrhythmias Alcohol = CNS depression Sun = photosensitivity
Bupropion • Wellbutrin • Zyban	**Insomnia, agitation, dry mouth, tremor, abnormal dreams, h/a, excess sweating, tachycardia, nausea, constipation, vomiting, dizziness, rhinitis, anorexia, blurred vision**, wt gain, seizures	MAO inhibitors = ↑ risk of toxicity Nicotine = hypertension Levodopa = ↑ risk of adverse reactions Sun = photosensitivity Prednisone or phenothiazine = ↑ risk of seizures

Antidepressants—cont'd

Indication = Depression, OCD, anxiety

Generic name (Brand names)	Adverse reactions (Most frequent are bolded)	Interactions
Fluoxetine* • Prozac	Nervousness, somnolence, insomnia, anxiety, drowsiness, h/a, tremor, dizziness, weakness, nausea, diarrhea, dry mouth, anorexia, akathisia	Beta blockers = heart block, bradycardia MAO inhibitors or St John's wort = serotonin syndrome Antipsychotics = ↑ concentration of antipsychotics (extrapyramidal signs) Warfarin = ↑ bleeding Alcohol = ↑ depression
Sertraline* • Zoloft	**Fatigue, h/a, tremor, dizziness, insomnia, somnolence, dry mouth, nausea, diarrhea, male sexual dysfunction,** suicidal behavior, akathisia	Benzodiazepines = ↑ effects MAO inhibitors, triptans, isoniazid, or St John's wort = serotonin syndrome Warfarin = ↑ bleeding

Exercise concerns: Improved motor performance following ischemic stroke

*Should not be taken with MAO inhibitors.

Decongestants, Antihistamines, & Bronchodilators

Indications = Bronchospasms, COPD, emphysema

Generic name (Brand names)	Adverse reactions (Most frequent are **bolded**)	Interactions
Albuterol • Proventil • Ventolin • Brethine	**Tremor, nervousness, h/a, hyperactivity, tachycardia, nausea, vomiting,** muscle cramps, hypocalcemia, cough, hyperglycemia	CNS stimulant = ↑ CNS effects MAO inhibitors or antidepressants = ↑ adverse CV effects Beta blockers = contraindicated, may cause bronchoconstriction
Pirbuterol • Maxair	Tremor, nervousness, dizziness, tachycardia, nausea, vomiting, cough, hyperglycemia	Beta blockers = contraindicated, may cause bronchoconstriction MAO inhibitors or antidepressants = ↑ effects
Salmeterol • Serevent discus	**Nasopharyngitis, URI,** h/a, tremor, nausea, nervousness, tachycardia, myalgia	Beta blockers = contraindicated, may cause bronchoconstriction MAO inhibitors or antidepressants = ↑ risk of severe CV effects

Exercise concerns: Diminished exercise performance; limited muscle endurance; systemic administration may ↑ hyperglycemia

Please note:

This list is not comprehensive and is subject to modification by various facilities to meet the needs of their patient population.

ā	before
A	assistance
AAA	abdominal aortic aneurysm
AAROM	active, assistive range of motion
Abd	abduction
ABG	arterial blood gases
ACL	anterior cruciate ligament
A.C.	before meals
Add	adduction
ADLs	activities of daily living
ad lib	as desired
AE	above elbow
AFib	atrial fibrillation
AFO	ankle foot orthosis
AK	above knee
AMA	against medical advice
amb	ambulation
ANS	autonomic nervous system
AP	anterior-posterior
APL	abductor pollicis longus
ARD	adult respiratory distress
AROM	active range of motion
ASA	aspirin
ASCVD	arteriosclerotic cardiovascular disease
ASIS	anterior superior iliac spine
ATFL	anterior talofibular ligament
A-V	arterio-venous
B	bilateral
BBB	bundle branch block
B&B	bowel & bladder
BE	below elbow
BID	twice daily
BK	below knee
BMI	body mass index
BMR	basal metabolic rate

BM	bowel movement
BOS	base of support
BP	blood pressure
BRP	bathroom privileges
BS	breath sounds
BUN	blood urea nitrogen
Bx	biopsy
c̄	with
Ca^{+1}	calcium
CA	cancer
CABG	coronary artery bypass graft
CAD	coronary artery disease
CBC	complete blood count
CC	chief complaint
CCE	clubbing, claudication, edema
CHF	congestive heart failure
CHI	closed head injury
CKC	closed kinetic chain
CN	cranial nerve
CNS	central nervous system
c/o	complaints of
CO	cardiac output
COPD	chronic obstructive pulmonary disease
CP	cerebral palsy
CP	chest pain
CPK	creatine phosphokinase
CPM	continuous passive motion
CPP	closed packed position
CPR	cardiopulmonary resuscitation
CSF	cerebral spinal fluid
CT	computed tomography
CTS	carpal tunnel syndrome
Ctx	cervical traction
CVA	cerebral vascular accident
CXR	chest x-ray
D/C	discharge
DDD	degenerative disc disease
DDX	differential diagnosis
DF	dorsiflexion
DIP	distal interphalangeal
DJD	degenerative joint disease

DM	diabetes mellitus
DNR	do not resuscitate
DOB	date of birth
DOE	dyspnea on exertion
DPT	diphtheria, pertussis, tetanus
DSD	dry sterile dressing
DTR	deep tendon reflexes
DVT	deep vein thrombosis
Dx	diagnosis
EAA	essential amino acids
BL	estimated blood loss
EEG	electroencephalogram
ECK, EKG	electrocardiogram
EMG	electromyogram
ENT	ear, nose, throat
EOMI	extra-ocular motion intact
EPB	extensor pollicis brevis
ER	external rotation
ESR	erythrocyte sedimentation rate
ETOH	ethyl alcohol
ev	eversion
Ex	exercise
Ext	extension
F	frequency
FAQ	full arc quads
FB	feedback
f/b	followed by
FCU	flexor carpi ulnaris
FDP	flexor digitorum profundus
FEV	forced expiratory volume
flex	flexion
FOOSH	fall on outstretched hand
FPL	flexor pollicis longus
FRC	functional residual capacity
FUO	fever of unknown origin
FVC	forced vital capacity
FWB	full weight bearing
Fx	fracture
f/u	follow-up
GB	gallbladder
GI	gastrointestinal

Grav. 1 . . . . .number of pregnancies (para = births)
GSW . . . . .gunshot wound
GTO . . . . .Golgi tendon organ
GTT . . . . .glucose tolerance test
GU . . . . .genitourinary
GXT . . . . .graded exercise tolerance
H&H . . . . .hematocrit & hemoglobin
HA . . . . .headache
Hct . . . . .hematocrit
HDL . . . . .high density lipoprotein
HEENT . . . . . . .head, ears, eyes, nose, throat
Hgb . . . . .hemoglubln
HIV . . . . .human immunodeficiency virus
HNP . . . . .herniated nucleus pulposus
H/O . . . . .history of
HOB . . . . .head of bed
HP . . . . .hot pack
HPI . . . . .history of present illness
HR . . . . .heart rate
HTN . . . . .hypertension
Hx . . . . .history
I . . . . .independent
I + D . . . . .incision & drainage
I + O . . . . .input & output
ICS . . . . .intercostal space
ICU . . . . .intensive care unit
IDDM . . . . .insulin dependent diabetes mellitus
I/E ratio . . . . . . .inspiratory/expiratory ratio
IM . . . . .intramuscular
inv . . . . .inversion
IP . . . . .interphalangeal joint
IPPB . . . . .Intermittent positive pressure breathing
IR . . . . .internal rotation
IRDM . . . . .insulin resistant diabetes mellitus
ITB . . . . .iliotibial band
IV . . . . .intravenous
JODM . . . . .juvenile onset diabetes mellitus
JRA . . . . .juvenile rheumatoid arthritis
JVD . . . . .jugular vein distension
KAFO . . . . .knee ankle foot orthosis
KUB . . . . .kidney, ureter, bladder

L	left
LBP	low back pain
LBQC	large-base quad cane
LCL	lateral collateral ligament
LDH	serum lactic dehydrogenase
LE	lower extremity
LKS	liver, kidney, spleen
LLB	long leg brace
LLC	long leg cast
LLQ	left lower quadrant
LMN	lower motor neuron
LMP	last menstrual period
LOC	loss of consciousness
LOS	length of stay
LP	lumbar puncture
LTG	long-term goal
LUQ	left upper quadrant
MAFO	molded ankle foot orthosis
MAL	midaxillary line
max	maximum
MCL	midclavicular line
MCL	medial collateral ligament
MCP	metacarpal phalangeal
MH	moist heat
min	minimum
MI	myocardial infarction
mm	muscle
MMR	measles, mumps, rubella
MMT	manual muscle test
mod	moderate
MOI	mechanism of injury
MRI	magnetic resonance imaging
MRSA	methicillin-resistant *Staph. aureus*
MS	multiple sclerosis
MTrP	myofascial trigger point
MTP	metatarsal phalangeal
MVA	motor vehicle accident
MWD	microwave diathermy
n/a	not applicable
N + V	nausea and vomiting
NAD	no acute distress

NCV	nerve conduction velocity
ng	nasogastric
NIDDM	noninsulin dependent diabetes mellitus
NKA	no known allergies
NKDA	no known drug allergies
nn	nerve
NPO	nothing by mouth
NSA	no significant abnormality
NSAID	nonsteroidal anti-inflammatory drug
NSR	normal sinus rhythm
NWB	non-weight bearing
O_2	oxygen
OA	osteoarthritis
OB	obstetrics
OKC	open kinetic chain
OOB	out of bed
OPP	open packed position
ORIF	open reduction, internal fixation
OT	occupational therapy
P + A	percussion and auscultation
P + PD	percussion + postural drainage
p	after
PA	posterior-anterior
PAC	premature atrial contraction
PAO2	alveolar oxygen
PaO2	peripheral arterial oxygen content
PAP	pulmonary artery pressure
PCL	posterior cruciate ligament
PD	postural drainage
PDR	Physicians' Desk Reference
PE	pulmonary embolus
PEEP	positive end expiratory pressure
PERLA	pupils equal reactive to light accommodation
PF	plantar flexion
PFT	pulmonary function tests
PID	pelvic inflammatory disease
PIP	proximal interphalangeal
PMH	past medical history
PNF	proprioceptive neuromuscular facilitation
P.O.	by mouth
POD	post-op day

PR	pulse rate
PRE	progressive resistive exercises
prn	as necessary
PROM	passive range of motion
PSIS	posterior superior iliac spine
pt	patient
PTB	patellar tendon bearing
PTFL	posterior talofibular ligament
PVC	premature ventricular contraction
PVD	peripheral vascular disease
PWB	partial weight bearing
Px	problem
q2°	every two hours
R	right
RA	rheumatoid arthritis
RBC	red blood count/cells
RCL	radial collateral ligament
RHD	rheumatic heart disease
RLQ	right lower quadrant
r/o	rule out
ROM	range of motion
ROS	review of systems
RPE	rate of perceived exertion
RR	respiratory rate
RUQ	right upper quadrant
RV	residual volume
Rx	treatment
s̄	without
S	supervision
S1	first heart sound
S2	second heart sound
SAQ	short arc quad
SBQC	small base quad cane
SC	straight cane
SC	sternoclavicular
SCI	spinal cord injury
SCM	sternocleidomastoid
SGOT	serum glutamic-oxalacetic transaminase
SI	sacroiliac
SLB	short leg brace
SLP	speech & language pathology

SLR	straight leg raises
SOAP	subjective, objective, assessment, plan
SOB	short of breath
s/p	status post
SPC	single-point cane
STG	short-term goal
SV	stroke volume
SWD	short wave diathermy
Sx	symptoms
S & S	signs and symptoms
TB	tuberculosis
TBI	traumatic brain injury
TENS	transcutaneous electrical neuromuscular stimulation
TE	therapeutic exercise
TFCC	triangular fibrocartilage complex
TFL	tensor fascia latae
TFM	transverse friction massage
THL	transverse humeral ligament
THR	total hip replacement
tid	three times daily
TKE	terminal knee extension
TKR	total knee replacement
TLC	total lung capacity
TMJ	temporomandibular joint
TOS	thoracic outlet syndrome
TPR	temperature, pulse, respiration
TPR	total peripheral resistance
TTP	tender to palpation
TTWB	toe touch weight bearing
TURP	transurethral resection of prostate
TV	tidal volume
TVH	total vaginal hysterectomy
Tx	treatment or traction
UCHD	usual childhood disease
UCL	ulnar collateral ligament
UE	upper extremity
ULNT	upper limb neurodynamic test(s)
UMN	upper motor neuron
URI	upper respiratory infection
US	ultrasound
UTI	urinary tract infection

UV	ultraviolet
VC	vital capacity
VMO	vastus medialis obliquus
V/O	verbal order
VPC	ventricular precontraction
VS	vital signs
VTO	verbal telephone order
WBAT	weight bearing as tolerated
WBC	white blood count/cells
WBTT	weight bearing to tolerance
WBQC	wide-base quad cane
WC	wheelchair
WFL	within functional limits
WNL	within normal limits
WP	whirlpool
XCT	chemotherapy
XRT	radiation therapy
yo	years old
1°	primary
2°	secondary
<	less than
>	greater than
↑	increase
↓	decrease
∥	parallel

Interpretation of Statistics

Sensitivity
- True positive rate
- Proportion of patients who have a pathology that the test identifies as positive
- **SnNout** = **Sn**sitivity, a **N**egative test rules **out** the diagnosis
- Calculation = $a/(a+c)$

Specificity (SpPin)
- True negative rate
- Proportion of patients who have a pathology that the test identifies as negative
- **SpPin** = **Sp**ecificity, a **P**ositive test rules **in** the diagnosis
- Calculation = $d/(b+d)$

Truth/Gold Standard			
	Present	**Absent**	
(+) Test	a	b	a + b
(–) Test	c	d	c + d
	a + c	b + d	a + b + c + d

Anatomy

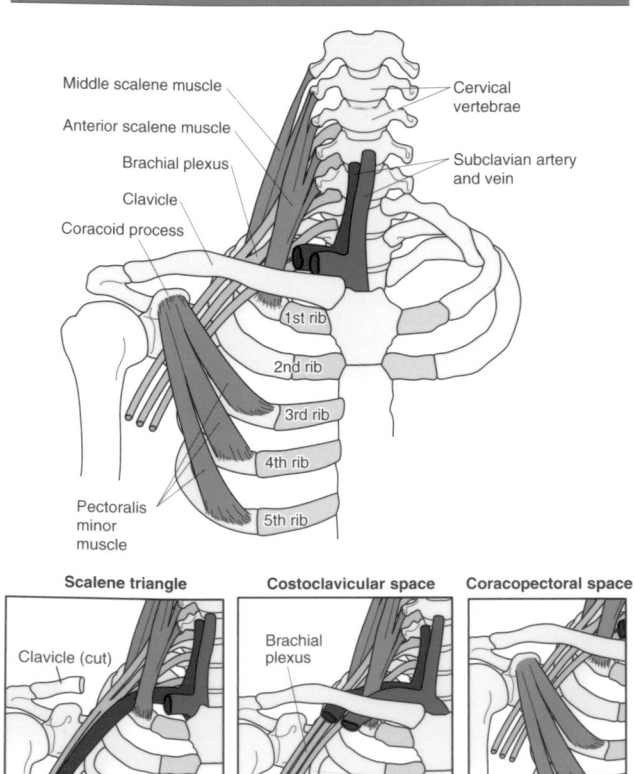

Middle scalene muscle

Anterior scalene muscle

Brachial plexus

Clavicle

Coracoid process

Cervical vertebrae

Subclavian artery and vein

1st rib

2nd rib

3rd rib

4th rib

5th rib

Pectoralis minor muscle

Scalene triangle

Clavicle (cut)

Costoclavicular space

Brachial plexus

Coracopectoral space

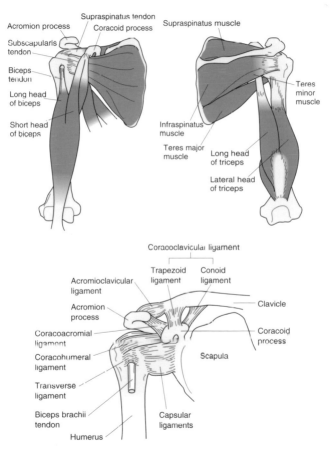

Acromion process
Supraspinatus tendon
Coracoid process
Supraspinatus muscle
Subscapularis tendon
Biceps tendon
Long head of biceps
Short head of biceps
Teres minor muscle
Infraspinatus muscle
Teres major muscle
Long head of triceps
Lateral head of triceps

Coracoclavicular ligament
Trapezoid ligament
Conoid ligament
Acromioclavicular ligament
Clavicle
Acromion process
Coracoacromial ligament
Coracoid process
Coracohumeral ligament
Scapula
Transverse ligament
Biceps brachii tendon
Capsular ligaments
Humerus

- **Pericarditis**
  - Sharp anterior chest & shoulder pain
  - ↑ temp, HR, RR
- **Cardiac ischemia**
  - Neck, jaw, left arm, & chest pain
  - SOB
  - Palpitations
  - ↑ BP
  - Syncope
- **Pulmonary pathology**
  - Neck, shoulder, mid-thorax pain
  - Cough
  - Fever
  - Shallow & ↑ RR
- **Sources of right shoulder/scapula pain**
  - Gallstones—8Fs
    - Fertile = 3rd trimester of pregnancy
    - Female
    - Fat
    - Forty
    - Fair
    - Food–fatty intake
    - Family history
    - Flatulence
  - Peptic ulcer (lateral border of scapula)
  - Diaphragm
  - Liver abscess, hepatic tumor
- **Sources of left shoulder pain**
  - MI
  - Diaphragm
  - Ruptured spleen
  - Pancreas

Shoulder Pain & Disability Index (SPADI)

Pain Scale: How severe is your pain?
0 = no pain ....10 = worse pain imaginable

■ At its worst?	0 1 2 3 4 5 6 7 8 9 10
■ When lying on the involved side?	0 1 2 3 4 5 6 7 8 9 10
■ Reaching for something on a high shelf?	0 1 2 3 4 5 6 7 8 9 10
■ Touching the back of your neck?	0 1 2 3 4 5 6 7 8 9 10
■ Pushing with the involved arm?	0 1 2 3 4 5 6 7 8 9 10

Disability Scale: How much difficulty do you have...
0 = no pain ....10 = worse pain imaginable

■ Washing your hair?	0 1 2 3 4 5 6 7 8 9 10
■ Washing your back?	0 1 2 3 4 5 6 7 8 9 10
■ Putting on an undershirt or pullover sweater?	0 1 2 3 4 5 6 7 8 9 10
■ Putting in a shirt that buttons down the front?	0 1 2 3 4 5 6 7 8 9 10
■ Putting on your pants?	0 1 2 3 4 5 6 7 8 9 10
■ Placing an object on a high shelf?	0 1 2 3 4 5 6 7 8 9 10
■ Carrying a heavy object of 10 pounds?	0 1 2 3 4 5 6 7 8 9 10
■ Removing something from your back pocket?	0 1 2 3 4 5 6 7 8 9 10

Pain Scale Score:
Disability Scale Score: **Total Score:**

Scoring: Summate the scores & divide by the number of scores possible. If an item is deemed not applicable, no score is calculated. Multiple the total score by 100. The higher the score, the greater the impairment.

Source: From Roach, KE, Buudimanmak, E, Songsirideg, N, Yongsuk, L. (1991).

Quick DASH (Disabilities of the Arm, Shoulder, & Hand)

Please rate your ability to do the following activities in the last week by circling the number below the appropriate response.	No Difficulty	Mild Difficulty	Moderate Difficulty	Severe Difficulty	Unable
1. Open a tight or new jar	1	2	3	4	5
2. Do heavy household chores (wash walls, floors)	1	2	3	4	5
3. Carry a shopping bag or briefcase	1	2	3	4	5
4. Wash your back	1	2	3	4	5
5. Use a knife to cut food	1	2	3	4	5
6. Recreational activities in which you take some force or impact through your arm, shoulder, or hand (golf, hammering, tennis, etc.)	1	2	3	4	5
	Not At All	Slightly	Moderately	Quite A Bit	Extremely
7. During the past week, to what extent has your arm, shoulder, or hand problem interfered with your normal social activities with family, friends, neighbors, or groups?	1	2	3	4	5

Continued

Quick DASH (Disabilities of the Arm, Shoulder, & Hand)—cont'd

	Not Limited	Slightly Limited	Moderately Limited	Very Limited	Unable
8 During the past week, were you limited in your work or other regular daily activities as a result of your arm, shoulder, or hand problem?	1	2	3	4	5

Please rate the severity of the following symptoms in the last week.

	None	Mild	Moderate	Severe	Extreme
9. Arm, shoulder, or hand pain	1	2	3	4	5
10. Tingling (pins & needles) in your arm, shoulder, or hand	1	2	3	4	5

	No Difficulty	Mild Difficulty	Moderate Difficulty	Severe Difficulty	So Difficult, I Can't Sleep
11. During the past week, how much difficulty have you had sleeping because of the pain in your arm, shoulder, or hand?	1	2	3	4	5

Quick DASH Score = [(sum of responses/number of responses) − 1] × 25

A Quick DASH score cannot be calculated if more than 1 item is not answered

Referral Patterns

Muscle Pain Referral Patterns

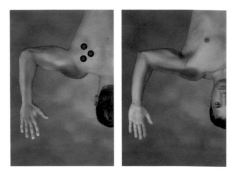

Infraspinatus

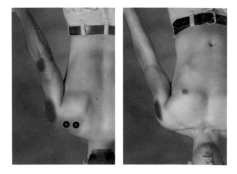

Supraspinatus

Subscapularis

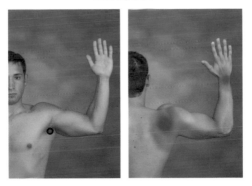

Teres Minor

Biceps Brachii

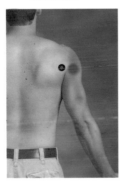

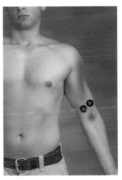

Palpation Pearls

Rotator Cuff Muscles

Supraspinatus With UE back in maximal extension & IR, palpate from the supraspinatus fossa to the tendon anterior to a-c joint	Infraspinatus In prone on elbows, palpate posterior-lateral of acromion (just inferior to inferior angle of acromion)
Subscapularis In side-lying, maneuver the relaxed UE to allow you to slide your thumb under the axillary/lateral border of the scapula	Teres Minor In prone on elbows, palpate just inferior to infraspinatus

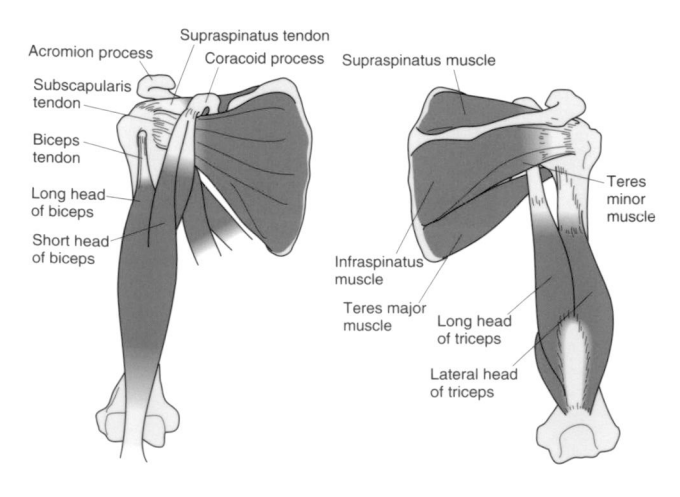

ROM

Rotational Lack

- Reach overhead (left figure) as far as possible down the back & mark the most inferior point of the fingers.
- Reach up the back as far as possible (right figure) & mark the most superior point of the fingers.
- Measure distance between the marks. This is the rotational lack.

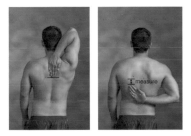

Apley Scratch Test for Quick Screen

3 components:

1. Hand to opposite shoulder
2. Hand behind back to opposite scapula
3. Hand behind back to inferior angle of opposite scapula

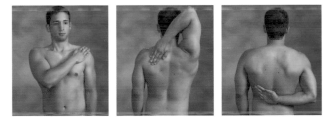

Capsular Patterns

Location of Capsular Tightness	Restrictions in Motion	Mobility Deficits
Posterior capsule	• ↓ Horizontal adduction, IR, & end range flexion • ↓ Posterior glide	• Weak ER • Poor scapular stability
Posterior-inferior capsule	• ↓ Elevation, IR, & horizontal adduction	
Posterior-superior capsule	• ↓ IR	
Anterior-superior capsule	• ↓ End range flexion & extension, ↓ ER & horizontal abduction	• Weak RC • (+) NTPT • Night pain
Anterior capsule	• ↓ Abduction, extension, ER, & horizontal adduction	

Osteokinematics of the Shoulder

Normal ROM	OPP	CPP	Normal End-feel(s)	Abnormal End-feel(s)
Elevation 165°–170° IR/ER 180° total Scapulo-Humeral Rhythm 2:1 (120°:60°)	55°–70° abduction 30° horizontal abduction	Maximal abduction & ER	*Flexion* = elastic, firm – bony contact *Abduction* = elastic *Scaption* = elastic *IR/ER* = elastic/firm *Horiz add* = soft tissue *Extension* = firm *Horiz abd* = firm/elastic	Empty = subacromial bursitis Hard capsular = frozen shoulder Capsular = ER > abduction > IR

Arthrokinematics for Shoulder Mobilization

Glenohumeral Joint			
	Concave surface: Glenoid fossa	*To facilitate elevation:* Humeral head spins posterior	*To facilitate abduction:* Humeral head rolls superior & glides inferior/posterior
		To facilitate IR: Humeral head rolls posterior & glides anterior	*To facilitate ER:* Humeral head rolls anterior & glides posterior
	Convex surface: Humeral head	*To facilitate horizontal adduction:* Humeral head rolls medial & glides lateral on glenoid	*To facilitate horizontal abduction:* Humeral head rolls lateral & glides medial on glenoid

Sternoclavicular Joint			
	Convex surface: Medial clavicle / Concave surface: Disk & manubrium	*To facilitate elevation:* Lateral clavicle rolls upward & medial clavicle glides inferior on disk & manubrium	*To facilitate depression:* Lateral clavicle rolls downward & medial clavicle glides superior on disk & manubrium
	Concave surface: Medial clavicle & disk / Convex surface: Manubrium	*To facilitate retraction:* Medial clavicle & disk rolls & glides posterior on manubrium	*To facilitate protraction:* Medial clavicle & disk rolls & glides anterior on manubrium

Force Couples of the Shoulder

- Elevation = trapezius, rhomboid, SA
- Upward rotation = upper/lower trapezius & SA
- Abduction = supraspinatus, subscapularis, & deltoid
- Downward rotation = lower trapezius, latissimus, & pectoralis minor
- Stabilization of the humeral head = RC & long head of biceps

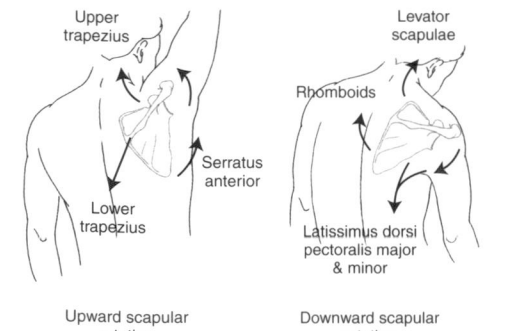

Upward scapular rotation

Downward scapular rotation

Neuromuscular Relationships of the Cervical Spine

Root	Nerve	Muscle	Sensation	Reflex
C3–4	Spinal accessory	Trapezius	⊘	⊘
C5	Dorsal scapular	Levator scapula Rhomboids	⊘	⊘
C5–6	Lateral pectoral	Pectoralis major Pectoralis minor	⊘	⊘
C5–6	Subscapular	Subscapular Teres major	⊘	⊘
C5–6	Long thoracic	Serratus anterior	⊘	⊘
C5–6	Suprascapular	Supraspinatus Infraspinatus	Top of shoulder	⊘
C5–6	Axillary	Deltoid Teres minor	Deltoid Anterior shoulder	⊘
C5–7	Musculocutaneous	Coracobrachialis Biceps & brachialis	Lateral forearm	Biceps
C5–T1	Radial	Triceps Wrist ext/finger flex	Dorsum of hand	Triceps
C6–7	Thoracodorsal	Latissimus dorsi	⊘	⊘

Nerve	Root	Muscle	Function
Radial	C5–8, T1	Anconeus, brachioradialis, ECRL, ECRB, extensor digitorum, APL, ECU, extensor indices, extensor digiti minimi	■ Weak supination, wrist extensors, finger flexors, thumb abductors ■ Weak grip due to loss of wrist stabilization
Median	C6–8, T1	Pronator teres, FCR, palmaris longus, FDS, FPL, pronator quadratus, thenar eminence, lateral 2 lumbricales	■ Weak pronation, wrist flexion & RD ■ Weak thumb flexion & abduction ■ Weak grip & pinch ■ Ape hand
Ulnar	C7–8, T1	FCU, palmaris brevis, hypothenar eminence, adductor pollicis, medial 2 lumbricales, interossei	■ Weak wrist flexion & UD ■ Weak 5th finger flexion ■ Weak finger abd/adduction ■ Benediction sign

Special Tests

Neural Tissue Provocation Tests

■ See Alerts/Alarms–page 14.

Shoulder Tests

EMPTY CAN TEST
Purpose: Test supraspinatus muscle
Position: Seated
Technique: Elevate UE 30°–45° in plane of the scapula with IR, resist elevation
Interpretation: + test = reproduction of pain &/or weakness
Statistics: Pain: sensitivity = 44%–100% & specificity = 50%–99%
Weakness: sensitivity = 77% & specificity = 68%

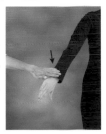

Source: From Gulick, D., 2008, page 108.

FULL CAN TEST
Purpose: Test supraspinatus muscle
Position: Seated
Technique: Elevate UE 30°–45° in plane of the scapula with ER, resist elevation
Interpretation: + test = reproduction of pain &/or weakness
Statistics: Pain: sensitivity = 66% & specificity = 64%
Weakness: sensitivity = 77% & specificity = 74%

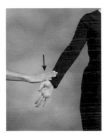

Source: From Gulick, D., 2008, page 109.

DROPPING SIGN
Purpose: Test infraspinatus muscle
Position: Seated
Technique: Shoulder at side with 45° of IR & 90° elbow flexion, resist ER
Interpretation: + test = reproduction of pain &/or weakness
Statistics: Sensitivity = 20%–42% & specificity = 69%–100%

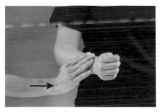

Source: From Gulick, D., 2008, page 109.

HORNBLOWER'S (PATTE TEST)

Purpose: Test teres minor muscle
Position: Seated
Technique: Shoulder in 90° abd & elbow flexed so that the hand comes to the mouth (blowing a horn)
Interpretation: + test = reproduction of pain &/or inability to maintain UE in ER

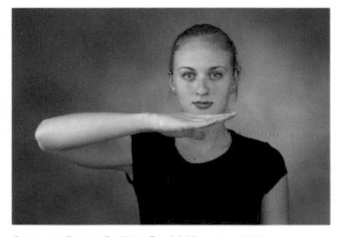

Source: From Gulick, D., 2008, page 110.

RENT SIGN

Purpose: Diagnosis RC tears
Position: Seated with UE in full ext & clinician's hand under the flexed elbow
Technique: Stand behind pt with fingertips in the anterior margin of the acromion; IR/ER UE & palpate for an eminence & a rent; compare bilaterally
Interpretation: + test = presence of a palpable defect in RC
Statistics: Sensitivity = 95% & specificity = 96%

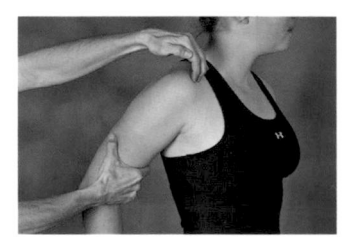

GERBER'S LIFT-OFF SIGN

Purpose: Test subscapularis muscle
Position: Seated
Technique: Hand in the curve of lumbar spine, resist IR
Interpretation: + test = reproduction of pain &/or weakness; inability to lift off
Statistics: Sensitivity = 62%–89% & specificity = 98%–100%; tears >75% are often required to produce a + test

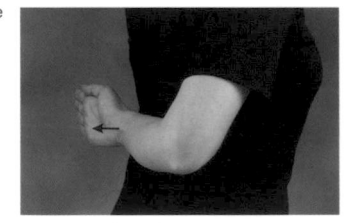

Source: From Gulick, D., 2008, page 110.

BELLY PRESS OR NAPOLEON SIGN

Purpose: Test subscapularis muscle
Position: Seated with hand on belly
Technique: Press the hand into belly
Interpretation: + test = reproduction of pain &/or inability to IR; substitution may result in UE elevation or wrist flexion
Statistics: Sensitivity = 25%–40% & specificity = 98%; tears >50% are often required to produce a + test

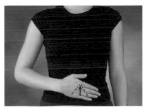

Source: From Gulick, D., 2008, page 111.

BEAR-HUG TEST

Purpose: Test subscapularis muscle
Position: Seated with palm of hand on opposite shoulder (elbow in front of body)
Technique: Resist IR by attempting to pull hand off the shoulder
Interpretation: + test = inability to hold the hand against the shoulder or weakness >20% of contralateral UE
Statistics: Sensitivity = 60% & specificity= 92%; tears of 30% can be detected with this test

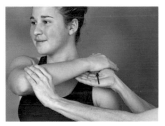

HAWKINS/KENNEDY TEST

Purpose: Test for impingement
Position: Seated
Technique: Place shoulder in 90° of flexion, slight horizontal adduction, & maximal IR
Interpretation: + test = shoulder pain due to impingement of supraspinatus between greater tuberosity against coracoacromial arch
Statistics: Sensitivity = 72%–92% & specificity = 25%–66%

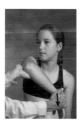

NEER'S TEST
Purpose: Test for impingement
Position: Seated
Technique: Passively take UE into full shoulder flexion with humerus in IR
Interpretation: + test = pain may be indicative of impingement of the supraspinatus or long head of the biceps
Statistics: Sensitivity = 68%–95% & specificity = 25%–68%

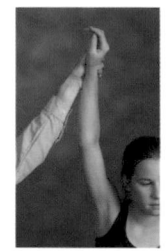

IMPINGEMENT RELIEF TEST
Purpose: Confirm impingement
Position: Seated
Technique: Perform an inferior glide of GH joint while elevating UE to Neer position
Interpretation: + test = reduction or no pain when elevation is accompanied by an inferior glide

SULCUS SIGN
Purpose: Assess for inferior instability or AC px
Position: Sitting with shoulder in neutral & elbow flexed to 90°
Technique: Palpate shoulder joint line while using proximal forearm as a lever to inferiorly distract humerus
Interpretation: + test = ≥ 1 finger-width gap @ the shoulder joint line or AC joint

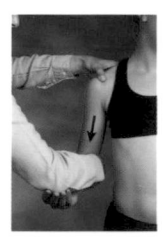

APPREHENSION TEST
Purpose: Assess for anterior instability
Position: Supine
Technique: Abduct the shoulder to 90° & then begin to ER
Interpretation: + test = pain or apprehension by the client to assume this position for fear of shoulder dislocation

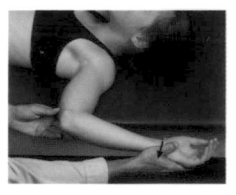

JERK TEST

Purpose: Assess posterior instability

Position: Sitting with UE in IR & flexed to 90°

Technique: Grasp client's elbow & load the humerus proximal while passively moving the UE into horizontal adduction

Interpretation: + test = a sudden jerk/clunk as the humeral head subluxes posteriorly; a second jerk/clunk may occur when the UE is returned to the abducted position

Statistics: Sensitivity = 73% & specificity = 90%

SPEED'S TEST

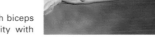

Purpose: Assess for biceps tendonitis or labrum problem

Position: Seated with shoulder elevated 75°–90° in the sagittal plane, elbow extended, & forearm supinated

Technique: Resist elevation

Interpretation: + test = pain with biceps tendonitis & sense of instability with labral px

Statistics: Sensitivity = 9%–100% & specificity = 61%–87%

BICEPS LOAD TEST

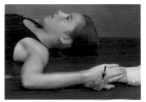

Purpose: Assess labrum

Position: Supine in 90°–120° of shoulder abduction & 90° of elbow flexion

Technique: Load the biceps by resisting elbow flexion/supination

Interpretation: + test = biceps tugs on labrum (SLAP) & reproduces pain

Statistics: Sensitivity = 91% & specificity – 97%

PAIN PROVOCATION TEST

Purpose: Assess labrum

Position: Supine in 90° shoulder abduction & 90° elbow flexion

Technique: Traction the biceps by passively taking the forearm into maximal pronation

Interpretation: + test = biceps will tug on labrum & reproduces the pain in the superior region of the joint line (superior labrum)

Statistics: Sensitivity = 17%–100% & specificity = 90%

CRANK TEST

Purpose: Assess labrum

Position: Seated with UE elevated to 160° & elbow flexed to 90°

Technique: Administer compression down the humerus while performing IR/ER

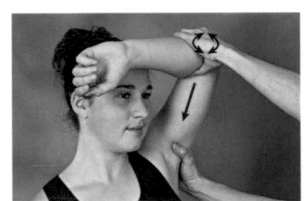

Interpretation: + test = pain or clicking

Statistics: Sensitivity = 39%–91% & specificity = 67%–93% (greater accuracy than MRI)

KIM TEST

Purpose: Assess labrum

Position: Seated with UE elevated to ~130° in the plane of the scapula & the elbow flexed to 90°

Technique: Apply a compressive force thru the humerus

Interpretation: + test = pain or clicking

Statistics: Sensitivity = 80%–82% & specificity = 86%–94%

O'BRIEN'S TEST

Purpose: Assess for labrum or AC joint problem

Position: Seated with UE in 90° of elevation, 10° of horiz add, & maximal IR (pronation)

Technique: Resist elevation in IR then repeat in ER (supination)

Interpretation: + test = pain in IR > ER; pain "inside" shoulder is labrum & pain "on top" of shoulder is AC

Statistics: Sensitivity = 47%–100% & specificity = 41%–98%

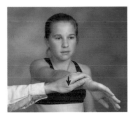
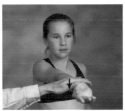

YERGASON'S TEST

Purpose: Assess THL

Position: Seated with shoulder in neutral, elbow flexed to 90°, & forearm supinated

Technique: Resist elbow flexion with supination

Interpretation: + test = pain with tenosynovitis; clicking or snapping with torn THL (with resistance from pronation to supination)

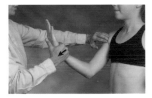

Statistics: Sensitivity = 9% 37% & specificity = 86%–96%

AC SHEAR TEST

Purpose: Assess for AC sprain

Position: Seated; UE at side

Technique: Clinician interlaces fingers & surrounds the AC joint; squeezing the hands together compresses the AC joint

Interpretation: + test = pain or excessive mov't is indicative of damage to the AC ligaments

Statistics: Sensitivity = 100% & specificity = 97%

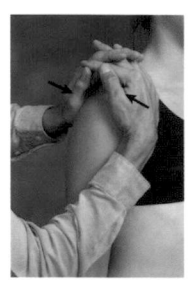

CORACOCLAVICULAR LIGAMENT TEST

Purpose: Assess CC ligament

Position: Side-lying on the unaffected side

Technique: Place affected UE behind back, palpate CC ligament while stabilizing clavicle; pulling inferior angle of scapula away from ribs to stress the conoid portion; pulling medial border of scapula away from the ribs stresses the trapezoid portion

Interpretation: + test = pain

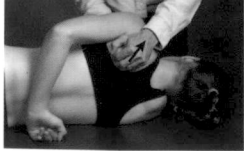
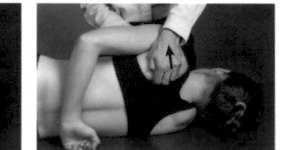

CROSS-BODY ADDUCTION TEST

Purpose: Assess for AC

Position: Seated

Technique: Shoulder flexed to 90°, horizontally adduct the UE

Interpretation: + test = pain @ AC joint

Statistics: Sensitivity = 100% & specificity = 97%

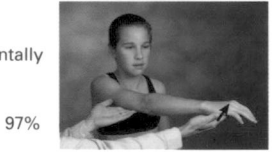

Thoracic Outlet Syndrome (TOS) Compression Sites

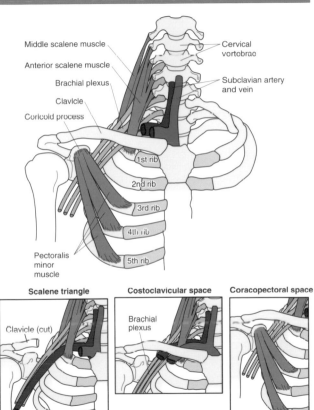

Middle scalene muscle

Anterior scalene muscle

Brachial plexus

Clavicle

Coricoid process

Cervical vortobrae

Subclavian artery and vein

1st rib

2nd rib

3rd rib

4th rib

5th rib

Pectoralis minor muscle

Scalene triangle

Clavicle (cut)

Costoclavicular space

Brachial plexus

Coracopectoral space

ADSON'S TEST

Purpose: Assess for TOS @ scalene triangle

Position: Seated

Technique: While palpating radial pulse, move UE into abd, ext, & ER, then client rotates head toward the involved side, takes a deep breath & holds it

Interpretation: + test = absent or diminished radial pulse with symptoms reproduced

Statistics: Specificity = 74%–89%

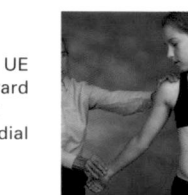

WRIGHT'S HYPERABDUCTION TEST

Purpose: Assess for TOS @ coracoid/rib & under pectoralis minor

Position: Seated

Technique: While palpating radial pulse, passively abduct UE to 180° in ER, have client take a deep breath & hold it

Interpretation: + test = absent or diminished radial pulse with symptoms reproduced

Statistics: Pulse: sensitivity = 70% & specificity = 53%
Pain: sensitivity = 90% & specificity = 29%

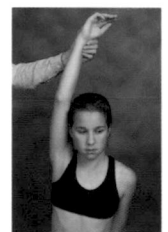

MILITARY BRACE (COSTOCLAVICULAR) TEST

Purpose: Assess for TOS @ 1st rib & clavicle

Position: Seated

Technique: While palpating radial pulse, retract shoulders into extension & abduction with the neck in hyperextension (exaggerated military posture)

Interpretation: + test = absent or diminished radial pulse or symptoms reproduced

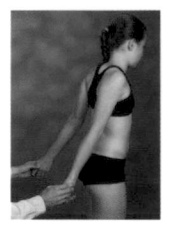

ALLEN'S TEST

Purpose: Assess for TOS @ pectoralis minor
Position: Seated
Technique: In 90° shoulder abduction & 90° elbow flexion, turn head away, take a deep breath & hold it
Interpretation: + test = absent or diminished radial pulse with symptoms reproduced

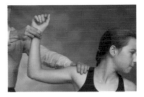

ROOS' TEST—Elevated Arm Stress Test (EAST)

Purpose: Assess for TOS
Position: Seated with UEs at 90° of shoulder abduction, ER, & elbow flexion.
Technique: Open & close hands repeatedly for 3 minutes
Interpretation: + test = reproduction of symptoms or sensation of heaviness of the UEs (record time of onset of symptoms)
Statistics: Sensitivity = 82%–84 & specificity = 30%–100%;

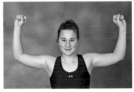

Combination of TOS tests	Sensitivity	Specificity
• Adson's + Wright's (pain)	79	76
• Adson's + Roos'	72	82
• Adson's + Hyperabd (pain)	72	88
• Adson's + Wright's (pulse)	54	94
• Wright's (pain) + Roos'	83	47
• Wright's (pain) + Hyperabd (pain)	83	50
• Wright's (pulse) + Hyperabd (pulse)	63	69

TOS—Differentiation Between Vascular & Neural Components

Vascular Components	Neural Components
■ (+) Adson's, Wright's, Allen's, Roos', military press test	■ Muscle weakness
■ Hand or arm edema	■ Pain with SB of C-spine
■ Discoloration or UE claudication	■ Sensory changes along a neurological distribution, i.e., radial or ulnar nerve
■ Change in skin temperature or texture	■ (+) Neural tissue provocation tests
■ Difference of >20 mm Hg in DBP between UEs	
■ Poor tolerance of cold & activity	

Differential Diagnosis

	TOS	C-disc	Shoulder	Cubital tunnel	Carpal tunnel
Pain	Intermittent neck, shoulder, arm	Sharp, constant neck & UE	Shoulder & proximal UE	Elbow & medial hand	Intermittent lateral hand
Headache	(+)	(–)	(–)	(–)	(–)
Numbness	Whole UE	Respective dermatome	No: common	Ulnar distribution	Median distribution
Edema	Possible	Normal	Normal	Normal	Normal
Color	May be abnormal	May be abnormal	Normal	Normal	May be abnormal
Provocation	UE elevation	Neck positions	Activity	Elbow pressure	Muscle cramping w/sustained grasp
Muscle strength	Weak triceps & RC	Specific myotomes	Weak RC	Ulnar innervations	Median innervations
(+) Tests	NTPT, Adson's, Allen's, military press, Roos'	Spurling's, NTPT	RC & impingement	Tinel's (elbow), NTPT	Phalens, CTS, Tinel's (wrist)

Pathology/Mechanism	Signs/Symptoms
Breast Cancer	■ Palpable mass/nodule in breast tissue ■ Nipple discharge, retraction, & local skin dimpling ■ Erythema, local rash ■ Confirmed with mammogram; biopsy
Thoracic Outlet Syndrome—results from compression of any one of many sites 2° postural or muscular imbalances or osseous anomalies. May be due to vascular (only 5%–10%) or neural compression; locations of compression include: sternocostovertebral space, scalene triangle, costoclavicular space, & coracopectoral space; most common in middle-aged female or after surgery **See "Neural vs Vascular Table" on page 76 for differential diagnosis.**	■ Kyphotic posture & forward head ■ Awakened @ night with pins & needles in hand ■ Poorly localized aching pain ■ Tenderness in the suprascapular fossa ■ Pain with carrying heavy objects ■ (+) Tests: NTPT, Adson's, Wright's, military brace, Roos' & Allen's ■ DBP > 20 mm Hg difference between arms ■ A/P x-ray needed to r/o cervical rib (very rare) ■ EMG results are controversial ■ Need to r/o CTS, radiculopathy, pronator syndrome
Glenohumeral Dislocation—anterior is most common (90%); mechanism is FOOSH	■ Prominent acromion, flattened shoulder silhouette, prominent humeral head ■ Injured posture: shoulder IR & slightly abducted, elbow flexed, forearm pronated, UE supported by contralateral limb ■ Sharp, stabbing pain, muscle guarding, humeral head is palpable anteriorly or inferiorly in the armpit ■ (+) Tests: Apprehension test & sulcus sign ■ X-ray—Hill-Sachs lesion may be visible in A/P view with UE in IR; Bankart lesion in Garth view ■ Need to r/o humeral neck fracture in elderly

Continued

Pathology/Mechanism	Signs/Symptoms
Clavicular Fracture—results from a fall on the shoulder or a direct blow to the clavicle	■ Can't raise arm ■ Visual deformity & TTP ■ Confirmed with x-ray
Acromioclavicular Sprain—may result from a fall on the acromion & FOOSH **See "Acromioclavicular Sprain Grades" on page 82.**	■ Pain & crepitus on palpation & visual deformity ■ (+) Tests: Cross body adduction, O'Brien's, AC shear, & sulcus/AC tx ■ Confirmed with bilateral A/P x-ray in ER with & without a 10–15 lb weight (stress films) ■ Need to r/o impingement
Labral Tear—may result from FOOSH, traction force on the shoulder, or a strong biceps contraction	■ Pain with IR & adduction ■ Weakness with abduction & flexion ■ Client reports a sense of instability ■ (+) Tests: Speed's test, O'Brien's, biceps load, pain provocation, & crank ■ Confirmed with CT or MRI; CT double contrast is more accurate than MRI
Subacromial Bursitis—chronic irritation resulting from trauma or poor biomechanics; may occur in middle-aged or older clients after an unusual bout of activity; hx of tendonitis	■ Swift onset of severe pain; localized to deltoid insertion ■ Noncapsular end-feel with no limitation in rotation (position of choice is adduction) ■ If bursitis exists in isolation (not common) then passive ROM is painful (noncontractile structure) & resistive motions are not painful (except in 50°–130° range where the contracting tendon compresses the bursa) ■ (+) Tests: Hawkins/Kennedy, Neer's & Impingement relief ■ Subacromial bursa warm & TTP (position UE into passive extension to palpate bursa) ■ Imaging is of little value unless calcification has occurred; need to r/o RC tear & impingement

Continued

Pathology/Mechanism	Signs/Symptoms
Bicipital Tendonitis—chronic irritation resulting from trauma or poor biomechanics Forward head contributes to abnormal scapulo-humeral rhythm	■ Pain ↑ @ night; TTP localized to biceps tendon @10° of IR (places tendon directly anterior & ~6 cm below acromion) ■ Active elevation results in a painful arc; crepitus ■ (+) Speed's test; (–) Yergason for click but painful ■ X-ray: bicipital groove view will reveal medial wall angle, spurs, degenerative changes; caudal tilt view will reveal spurring ■ Often associated with RC impingement
Calcific Tendonitis—cyclic problem of calcification = deposition & resorption with unknown etiology (may be related to tissue hypoxia) Occurs in ♀ > ♂; R > L; 40–50 yo	■ ↓ ROM with painful arc 70°–110° & sensation of catching when going thru ROM ■ (+) Speed's test ■ *During deposition:* chronic mild-moderate discomfort, throbbing unrelieved by rest ■ *During resorption:* acute ↑ in pain; sharp & localized ■ Confirmed by A/P film in neutral ■ Need to r/o impingement & adhesive capsulitis
Rotator Cuff Strain—results from mechanical compression OR tensile overload (eccentric microtears); partial thickness tears occur 25–40 yo & full thickness tears >60 yo RC has limited resiliency for self-repair *Contributing factors:* Posture—forward head influences GH alignment Antero-inferior capsule tightness = ↓ ER Posterior capsule tightness = ↑ superior & anterior translation of humeral head	■ Painful arc with UE motion; night pain; deep ache ■ Crepitus ■ Weakness: abduction +/or ER; protective shoulder hike ■ (+) Special tests depending on muscle involved—empty/full can (supraspinatus), lift-off or belly press/Napoleon (subscapularis), hornblowers (teres minor), dropping sign (infraspinatus); (+) O'Brien's test ■ Strength imbalance (ER MMT should be 60%–70% of IR)

Continued

Pathology/Mechanism	Signs/Symptoms
	■ X-ray may be normal with small tears; partial tears = superior humeral displacement may be evident with ER; full-thickness tear = narrowed acromiohumeral interval & osteophytes on anterior/inferior acromion ■ Diagnostic ultrasound is reliable for tears > 1 cm ■ Arthrography with contrast = Geyser's sign (painful) ■ MRI is noninvasive but CT double contrast is more accurate than MRI for full thickness RC tears
Supraspinatus Impingement—results from a progressive loss of humeral depressor mechanism (infraspinatus, subscapularis, teres minor, & long head of biceps) 2° overuse, cervical px, postural px, abnormal biomechanics, or structural px with acromion Microtrauma results from IR during overhead tennis stroke, swim, throwing; shoulder instability; tight pectoralis minor or weak lower trap & SA allows tipping of scapula with shoulder elevation to ↓ subacromial space to impingement	■ Pain (especially when sleeping on affected side) ■ Painful arc (60°–120° of elevation) ■ Pain & weakness in supraspinatus & biceps ■ "Catching" with flexion in IR ■ Pain referral pattern = deltoid insertion & anterior/proximal humerus ■ Little to no TTP ■ ROM ↓ IR & horizontal adduction ■ Posterior capsule tightness; pain with PROM ■ (+) Tests: Neer's, Hawkins-Kennedy, Speed's, empty/full can, & Yocum ■ X-rays may reveal ↓ joint space, arthritis, calcific tendonitis, hooked acromion; early dx is via MRI ■ Should r/o RC tear, TOS, labral tear, & calcific tendonitis
Coracoid Impingement—subacromial arch boundaries = acromion, coracoid, & coracoacromial ligament; houses supraspinatus, long head of biceps, subacromial bursa, coracohumeral ligament; hooked acromion; results from repetitive tasks with UE IR; poor posture	■ Dull pain in the front of the shoulder provoked by flexion & IR OR abduction & IR ■ Weak downward rotators of scapula ■ Forward head & kyphosis influences GH alignment ■ (+) Tests: Neer's, Hawkins-Kennedy, & impingement relief

Continued

Pathology/Mechanism	Signs/Symptoms
	■ X-ray will detect ↓ joint space & hooked acromion ■ Should r/o RC tear, TOS, labral tear, & calcific tendonitis
Adhesive Capsulitis—self-limiting disorder of unknown etiology; high incidence in DM & associated with old Colles fx; proliferation of collagen results in thickening of inferior capsule & loss of capsular folds; most common in ♀ 40–70 yo **See "Stages & Presentation of Adhesive Capsulitis" on page 83.**	■ Pain radiating to elbow; night pain ■ Kyphotic posture, shoulder hiking, low-grade inflammatory response ■ Empty end-feel; ↓ accessory movement ■ ROM limitations: ER > abduction > IR & reverse scapulohumeral rhythm (scapular 2: humeral 1) ■ Unable to sleep on affected side; MTrP subscapularis ■ Contrast arthrography = 50% reduction in shoulder joint volume (5–10 mL instead of 20–30 mL); plain films only reveal osteoporosis 2° to disuse atrophy

Acromioclavicular Sprain Grades

Grade	Presentation
Normal	Acromion to clavicle space should be ~ 0.3–0.8 cm Inferior clavicle to coracoid distance should be 1.0–1.3 cm
1st degree injury	AC joint space >0.8 cm & pain with horizontal adduction & elevation; (+) AC shear test
2nd degree injury	AC joint space 1.0–1.5 cm & CC distance increased by 25%–50%
3rd degree injury	AC joint space >1.5 cm & CC distance increased by >50% with a step deformity

Stages & Presentation of Adhesive Capsulitis

Stage	Clinical Findings	Arthroscopic Findings	Intervention
I—Freezing	• Continual increase in pain (before end-range) • ↓ A & PROM	Erythematous, fibrinous pannus over the synovium in the axillary fold	*Least aggressive:* • Modalities • Gentle AROM–Codman's • Grade I & II mobilizations
II—Frozen	• ↓ pain • ↓ A & PROM • Impaired GH accessory & physiological mov't • Impaired SH rhythm	Thickened synovium with adhesions developing across the folds	*Moderately aggressive:* • Modalities • AROM • Gentle PROM • Grade III & IV mobilizations
III—Thawing	• Pain with stretching only, ↑ accessory & physiologic motion, return of SH rhythm & ADLs	Loss of joint space, humeral head is compressed against glenoid, & axillary fold is reduced by 50%	*Most aggressive:* • Modalities • PROM • Grade III & IV mobilizations • PREs

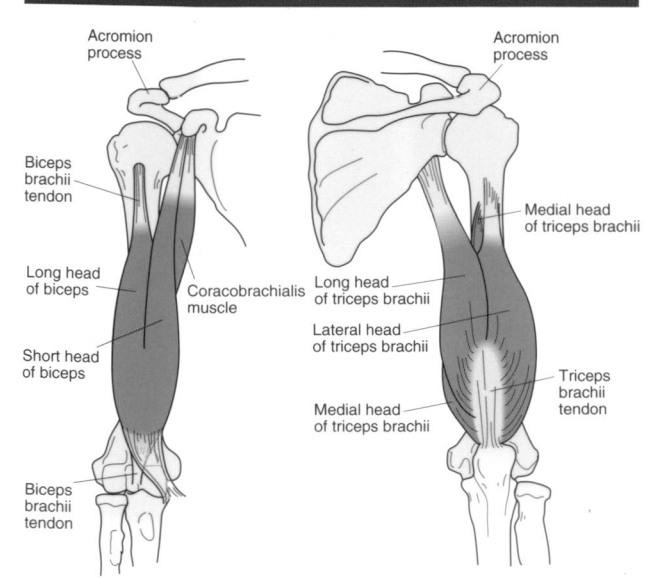

85

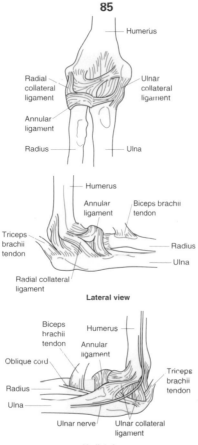

Lateral view

Medial view

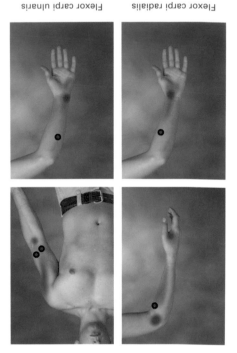

Referral Patterns

Muscle Pain Referral Patterns

Flexor carpi ulnaris

Flexor carpi radialis

Biceps brachii

Brachioradialis

Muscle Pain Referral Patterns

Extensor carpi ulnaris

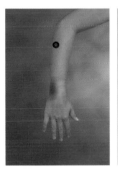

Extensor carpi radialis longus

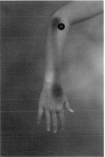

Extensor carpi radialis brevis

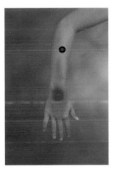

- Carrying angle of the elbow
  - 10°–15° valgus in ♀
  - 5°–10° valgus in ♂

Palpation Pearls

Wrist Extensor Muscles

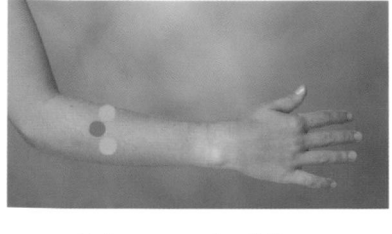

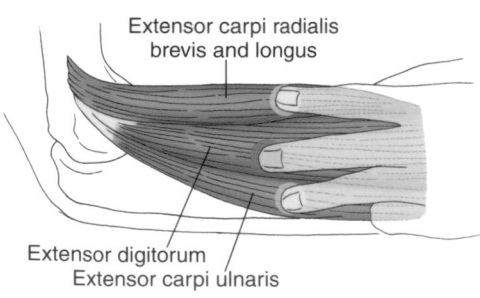

Extensor carpi radialis
brevis and longus

Extensor digitorum
Extensor carpi ulnaris

Wrist Flexor Muscles

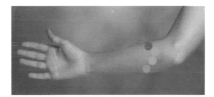

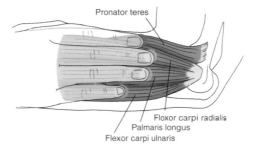

Pronator teres

Floxor carpi radialis
Palmaris longus
Flexor carpi ulnaris

Osteokinematics of the Elbow

Normal ROM		OPP	CPP	Normal End-feel(s)	Abnormal End-feel(s)
Flexion >135°	Humero-ulnar	70° flex 10° sup	full ext full sup	Flexion = soft tissue or bony approximation Extension = bony approximation	Boggy = joint effusion Capsular = flex > ext
	Humero-radial	full ext full sup	90° flex 5° sup		
Pronation & Supination 80°–90° each	Superior radio-ulnar	70° flex 35° sup	5° sup	Supination = ligamentous Pronation = bony approximation or ligamentous	Capsular = pronation & supination equally limited

Arthrokinematics for Elbow Mobilization

Humero-ulnar	Concave surface: Trochlear notch of ulna Convex surface: Trochlea of humerus	To facilitate flexion: OKC = radius & ulna roll & glide anterior & medial on humerus	To facilitate extension: OKC = radius & ulna roll & glide posterior & lateral on humerus
Humero-radial	Concave surface: Radial head Convex surface: Capitulum of humerus		
Superior/ proximal radio-ulnar	Concave surface: Radial notch of ulna Convex surface: Radial head	To facilitate pronation: Radius spins medial & glides anterior on ulna	To facilitate supination: Radius spins laterally on ulna

Strength & Function

Brachial Plexus–Roots, Muscles, & Function

Nerve	Root	Muscle	Functional Deficits
Median	C6–8, T1	Pronator teres, FCR, palmaris longus, FDS, FPL, pronator quadratus, thenar eminence, lateral 2 lumbricales	■ Weak pronation, wrist flexion, & RD ■ Weak thumb flexion & abduction ■ Weak grip & pinch ■ Ape hand
Ulnar	C7–8, T1	FCU, palmaris brevis, hypothenar eminence, adductor pollicis, medial 2 lumbricales, interossei	■ Weak wrist flexion & UD ■ Weak 5th finger flexion ■ Weak finger abd/adductor ■ Benediction sign
Radial	C5–8, T1	Anconeus, brachioradialis, ECRL, ECRB, extensor digitorum, APL, ECU, extensor indicis, extensor digiti minimi	■ Weak supination, wrist extension, finger flexion, thumb abduction ■ Weak grip due to loss of wrist stabilization

Brachial Plexus–Roots, Muscles, Deficits, & Deformities

Nerve & Root	Muscles	Functional Deficits	Postural Deformity
Radial C5–8 T1	Anconeus, brachioradialis, ECRL, ECRB, extensor digitorum, APL, ECU, extensor indicis, extensor digiti minimi	■ Weak supination, wrist ext, finger flex, thumb abd ■ Weak grip due to loss of wrist stabilization	
Median C6–8 T1	Pronator teres, FCR, palmaris long, FDS, FPL, pronator quadratus, thenar eminence, lateral 2 lumbricales	■ Weak pronation, wrist flex, & RD ■ Weak thumb flex & abd ■ Weak grip & pinch ■ Ape hand	
Ulnar C7–8 T1	FCU, palmaris brevis, hypothenar eminence, adductor pollicis, medial 2 lumbricales, interossei	■ Weak wrist flex & UD ■ Weak 5th finger flex ■ Weak finger abd/add ■ Benediction sign (Bishop's deformity)	

Source for top figure: From Levangie, PK, & Norkin, CC. Joint Structure & Function: A Comprehensive Analysis. 3rd ed. FA Davis, Philadelphia, 2001, page 107.

Special Tests

Neural Tissue Provocation Tests

See Alerts/Alarms page 14.

Elbow Tests

VARUS STRESS
Purpose: Assess LCL/RCL
Position: Elbow slightly flexed, humerus stabilized proximal to elbow (testing in prone enhances stabilization)
Technique: Apply a varus force to joint line to stress LCL
Interpretation: + test = pain or joint gapping/instability

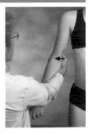

VALGUS STRESS
Purpose: Assess MCL/UCL
Position: Elbow slightly flexed, humerus stabilized proximal to elbow (testing in prone enhances stabilization)
Technique: Apply a valgus force to joint line to stress MCL
Interpretation: + test = pain or joint gapping/instability

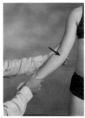

ACTIVE ELBOW TEST
Purpose: Assess MCL/UCL
Position: Sitting with shoulder in 90° abduction & elbow in full flexion
Technique: Apply a valgus force to elbow to take shoulder into full ER & while maintaining valgus force, quickly extend the elbow
Interpretation: + test = medial elbow pain between 120° & 70° of elbow motion

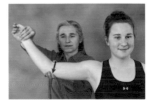

PRONATOR TERES TEST

Purpose: Assess for median nerve entrapment
Position: UE relaxed in supported position
Technique: Resist pronation of forearm
Interpretation: + test = pain along the palmar aspect of digits 1, 2, & 3 (median nerve distribution)

MILL'S TEST

Purpose: Assess for lateral epicondylitis
Position: UE relaxed, elbow extended
Technique: Passively stretch into wrist flexion & pronation
Interpretation: + test = pain @ lateral epicondyle or proximal musculotendinous junction of wrist extensors

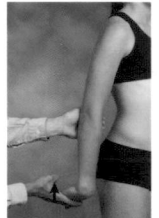

COZEN'S SIGN

Purpose: Assess for lateral epicondylitis
Position: UE relaxed, elbow extended
Technique: Resist supination & wrist extension OR resist middle finger extension (extensor digitorum)
Interpretation: + test = pain @ lateral epicondyle or proximal musculo-tendinous junction of wrist extensors

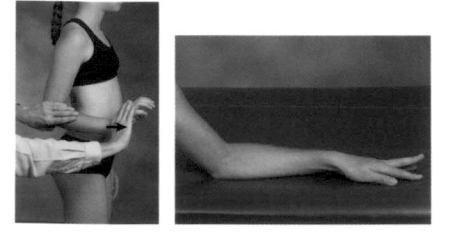

PASSIVE TEST
Purpose: Assess for medial epicondylitis
Position: UE relaxed, elbow extended
Technique: Stretch into wrist extension & supination
Interpretation: + test = pain @ medial epicondyle or proximal musculotendinous junction of wrist flexors

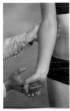

RESISTIVE TEST
Purpose: Assess for medial epicondylitis
Position: UE relaxed, elbow extended
Technique: Resist pronation & wrist flexion
Interpretation: + test = pain @ medial epicondyle or proximal musculotendinous junction of wrist flexors

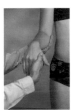

WARTENBERG'S TEST
Purpose: Assess for ulnar nerve entrapment
Position: UE relaxed in supported position
Technique: Resist 5th digit adduction
Interpretation: + test – weakness of 5th digit adductors

POSTEROLATERAL or ROTATORY INSTABILITY
Purpose: Assess for elbow instability
Position: Elbow extended
Technique: Apply an axial load with a valgus stress & supination
Interpretation: + test = elbow subluxes with extension & relocates with flexion

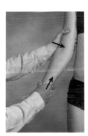

TINEL'S TEST

Purpose: Assess ulnar nerve

Position: Elbow in slight flexion

Technique: Tap groove between olecranon & lateral epicondyle

Interpretation: + test = pain & tingling in the distribution of ulnar nerve (4th & 5th digits)

Statistics: Sensitivity = 28% & specificity = 23%

Differential Diagnosis	
Pathology/Mechanism	**Signs/Symptoms**
Elbow Dislocation (posterior)—common in children & young adults due to a FOOSH	■ Pain, inability to flex elbow, deformity, tenderness ■ Confirmed by x-ray ■ Need to r/o fx & check distal pulses ■ **<u>Beware</u>** of possible development of myositis ossificans in brachialis muscle
Radial Head Subluxation—common in children 2–4 yo resulting from a child being picked up or swung by the hand or forearm & creating a distraction force	■ Child will autosplint in pronation & flexion ■ Radial head is TTP & child reports wrist discomfort from ↑ pressure from radial head being displaced distally ■ X-ray if fx is suspected ■ Reduction process = thumb in cubital fossa to serve as a fulcrum, supinate & flex the forearm (will "pop" in)
MCL Sprain—elongation/tear of ligament(s); common in throwing athletes 2° valgus stress	■ Acute trauma may experience a "pop" ■ TTP @ medial joint line ■ Valgus instability ■ Confirm with MRI; need to r/o avulsion

Continued

Pathology/Mechanism	Signs/Symptoms
Olecranon Bursitis—"student's elbow"—may result from direct trauma or repetitive UE activity	■ Defined mass at the olecranon that is warm, thick, & "gritty" to palpation ■ ↓ Elbow extension with nonspecific TTP ■ MRI used to confirm
Humerus & Radial Head Fracture—results from a FOOSH	■ Need to r/o avulsion & RCL/UCL sprain ■ AP & lateral plain film to confirm
Ulnar Neuritis—results from repetitive activity or trauma	■ Weak UD, 4th & 5th finger flexion ■ Pain with elbow flexion ■ (+) Tests: Tinel's, Wartenberg's, & NTPT ■ Paresthesia into forearm & 5th digit ■ Need to r/o C-spine pathology & TOS
Osteochondritis Dissecans—results from repetitive valgus stresses, such as throwing or gymnastics or frequent compressive forces (avascularity of subchondral bone = Panner's disease)	■ Confirm with MRI ■ Lateral elbow pain with ↓ elbow extension ■ Catching/locking of the elbow; pain with UE WB ■ Crepitus with pronation/supination ■ X-ray, MRI, CT are helpful in identifying a loose body
Reflex Sympathetic Dystrophy or Complex Regional Pain Syndrome—may be linked to previous trauma but a large percentage have no precipitating factor	■ Abnormal reflexes; varied manifestations of pain, burning, & edema ■ Nerve adhesions = (+) NTPT (movement is painful) ■ Vasomotor instability & trophic changes span from warm, redness over dorsum of MP & IP joints, & excessive moisture to cold temperature, pallor, & dryness of hand ■ Osteoporosis ■ MRI may or may not be helpful

Continued

Pathology/Mechanism	Signs/Symptoms
Avulsion/Stress Fracture of Medial Epicondyle = "Little League Elbow"—2° repetitive throwing motion; seen in teenagers with acceleration of UE with elbow flexion & valgus stress	■ Progressive pain & TTP @ medial epicondyle ■ ↓ ROM ■ (+) Valgus stress test ■ Confirm with x-ray or MRI
Medial Epicondylitis—"Golfer's Elbow"—insidious onset 2° to repetitive forces on the elbow; effects pronator teres & FCR	■ Pain with resisted wrist flexion & UD &/or passive stretching into wrist extension & supination with RD ■ TTP at proximal musculotendinous jctn of wrist flexors & pronators ■ (+) Passive & resistive tests ■ MRI may confirm diagnosis & r/o fx or avulsion
Lateral Epicondylitis—"Tennis Elbow"—overuse or microtrauma to lateral musculature; may result from a small racket grip, a racket that is too stiff or heavy, or a small sweet spot; usually involves ECRB	■ Morning stiffness ■ Pain with resisted wrist extension, supination, & RD *OR* passive stretching into wrist flexion, pronation, & UD ■ (+) Tests: Cozen's & Mill's ■ TTP at proximal musculotendinous junction of wrist extensors & supinators ■ MRI may confirm diagnosis & r/o fx or avulsion

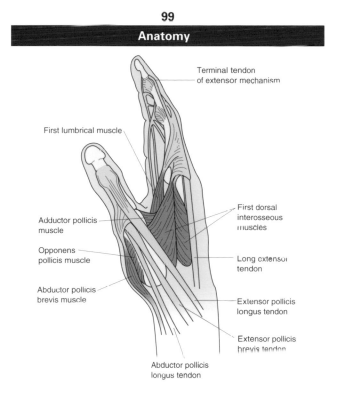

Terminal tendon of extensor mechanism

First lumbrical muscle

First dorsal interosseous muscles

Adductor pollicis muscle

Opponens pollicis muscle

Long extensor tendon

Abductor pollicis brevis muscle

Extensor pollicis longus tendon

Extensor pollicis brevis tendon

Abductor pollicis longus tendon

Medical Red Flags

- Digital clubbing
  - Acute pulmonary abscess
  - Pulmonary malignancy
  - Cirrhosis
  - Heart disease
  - Ulcerative colitis
  - COPD
- Spoon nails
  - Anemia
  - Thyroid px
  - Syphilis
  - Rheumatic fever
- Eggshell nails = thinning/semitransparent = syphilis
- Nail inflammation, infection, biting
- Paresthia in glove distribution
  - DM
  - Lead/mercury poisoning
- Hand tremor
  - Parkinsonism
  - Hypoglycemia
  - Hyperthyroidism
  - ETOH
  - MS
- Causes of CTS
  - Hx of statins (cholesterol drugs: Zocor or Lipitor)
  - Liver disease
  - Hypothyroidism
  - Gout
  - DM
  - Pregnancy/oral contraceptives
  - B_6 vitamin deficiency

Toolbox Tests

Rheumatoid Hand Functional Disability Scale That Assesses Functional Handicap

Answer the following questions regarding your ability without the help of any assistive devices:

Answers to the questions:	0 = Yes, without difficulty 1 = Yes, with a little difficulty 2 = Yes, with some difficulty 3 = Yes, with much difficulty 4 = Nearly impossible to do 5 = Impossible	
■ Can you hold a bowl?		
■ Can you seize a full bottle & raise it?		
■ Can you hold a plate full of food?		
■ Can you pour liquid from a bottle into a glass?		
■ Can you unscrew the lid from a jar opened before?		
■ Can you cut meat with a knife?		
■ Can you prick things well with a fork?		
■ Can you peel fruit?		
■ Can you button your shirt?		
■ Can you open & close a zipper?		
■ Can you squeeze a new tube of toothpaste?		
■ Can you hold a toothbrush efficiently?		
■ Can you write a short sentence with a pencil or ordinary pen?		
■ Can you write a letter with a pencil or ordinary pen?		
■ Can you turn a round door knob?		
■ Can you cut a piece of paper with scissors?		
■ Can you pick up coins from a table top?		
■ Can you turn a key in a lock?		
Score:		

Scoring: Summate all scores—the higher the score, the greater the disability

Source: From Duruoz, MT, Poiradeau, S, Fermanian, J, et al. Journal of Rheumatology, 23:7, 1996.

Patient Rated Wrist Evaluation

Rate the average amount of pain/difficulty you have had in your wrist over the past week by circling the number from 0 (no pain or difficulty) to 10 (the worse pain you have ever experienced or you could not do the task).

PAIN:

■ At rest	0 1 2 3 4 5 6 7 8 9 10
■ When doing a task with repeat wrist movement	0 1 2 3 4 5 6 7 8 9 10
■ When lifting a heavy object	0 1 2 3 4 5 6 7 8 9 10
■ When it is at its worst	0 1 2 3 4 5 6 7 8 9 10
■ How often do you have pain?	0 1 2 3 4 5 6 7 8 9 10

FUNCTION—SPECIFIC ACTIVITIES:

■ Turn a door knob using my affected hand	0 1 2 3 4 5 6 7 8 9 10
■ Cut meat using a knife in my affected hand	0 1 2 3 4 5 6 7 8 9 10
■ Fasten buttons on my shirt	0 1 2 3 4 5 6 7 8 9 10
■ Use my affected hand to push up from a chair	0 1 2 3 4 5 6 7 8 9 10
■ Carry a 10-lb object in my affected hand	0 1 2 3 4 5 6 7 8 9 10
■ Use bathroom tissue with my affected hand	0 1 2 3 4 5 6 7 8 9 10

FUNCTION—USUAL ACTIVITIES:

■ Personal care activities (dressing, washing)	0 1 2 3 4 5 6 7 8 9 10
■ Household work (cleaning)	0 1 2 3 4 5 6 7 8 9 10
■ Work (your job or everyday work)	0 1 2 3 4 5 6 7 8 9 10
■ Recreational activities	0 1 2 3 4 5 6 7 8 9 10

Score:

Pain subscale:	/50
Function subscale (total divided by 2):	/50
Total PRWE score:	/100

Scoring: Each section can be summated individually or the total scores can be calculated & scored as percentages. For either method, the higher the score, the poorer the outcome.

Source: Adapted from Lewis, C, Wilk, K, Wright, R. The Orthopedic Outcomes Toolbox. Virginia: Learn Publications.

Severity of Symptoms & Functional Status in Carpal Tunnel Syndrome

The following questions refer to your symptoms for a typical 24-hour period during the past 2 weeks. Circle 1 answer for each question.

How severe is the hand or wrist pain you have at night? 1. No pain 2. Mild pain 3. Moderate pain 4. Severe pain 5. Very severe pain	How often did hand or wrist pain wake you up during a typical night in the past 2 weeks? 1. Never 2. 1 time 3. 2–3 times 4. 4–5 times 5. More than 5 times	Do you typically have pain in your hand or wrist during the daytime? 1. No pain 2. Mild pain 3. Moderate pain 4. Severe pain 5. Very severe pain
How often do you have hand or wrist pain during the daytime? 1. Never 2. 1 time 3. 2–3 times 4. 4–5 times 5. More than 5 times	How long, on average, does an episode of pain last during the daytime? 1. Never have pain 2. Less than 10 minutes 3. 10–60 minutes 4. More than 60 minutes 5. Constantly	Do you have numbness (loss of sensation) in your hand? 1. No numbness 2. Mild numbness 3. Moderate numbness 4. Severe numbness 5. Very severe numbness
Do you have weakness in your hand or wrist? 1. No weakness 2. Mild weakness 3. Moderate weakness 4. Severe weakness 5. Very severe weakness	Do you have tingling sensation in your hand? 1. No tingling 2. Mild tingling 3. Moderate tingling 4. Severe tingling 5. Very severe tingling	How severe is the numbness or tingling at night? 1. No numbness/tingling 2. Mild numbness/tingling 3. Moderate numbness/tingling 4. Severe numbness/tingling 5. Very severe numbness/tingling
How often did hand numbness or tingling wake you up during a typical night in the past 2 weeks? 1. Never 2. 1 time 3. 2–3 times 4. 4–5 times 5. More than 5 times	Do you have difficulty with the grasping & use of small objects, such as keys or pencils? 1. No difficulty 2. Mild difficulty 3. Moderate difficulty 4. Severe difficulty 5. Very severe difficulty	*Scoring:* Summate the scores & divide by 11. The higher the mean score, the more severe the impairment. **Score:** _____

Source: From Levine, et al., Journal of Bone and Joint Surgery, 75A(11): 1585-1592, 1993.

Muscle Pain Referral Patterns

Flexor digitorum

Pronator teres

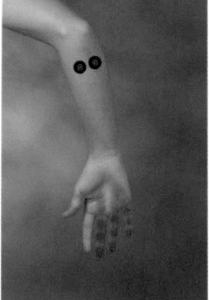

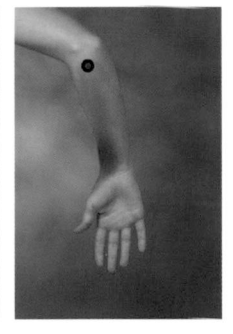

Flexor pollicis longus

1st dorsal interossei

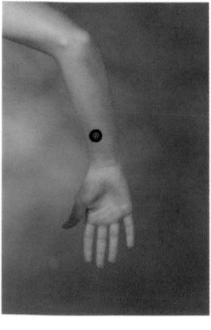

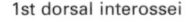

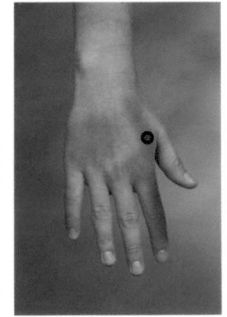

Abductor digiti minimi
& 2nd dorsal interossei

Opponens pollicis

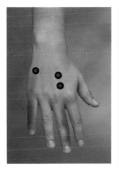

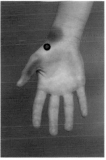

Adductor pollicis

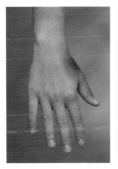

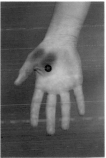

Pathologic Observations

Swan neck   Mallet

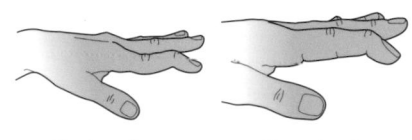

Boutonnière   Dupuytren's

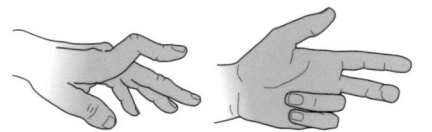

- When fist is clenched, all fingers should point to the scaphoid
- Heberden node = DJD of DIP
- Bouchard node = DJD of PIP
- Swan neck = MCP & DIP flexion with PIP hyperextension
- Boutonnière = MCP & DIP extension with PIP flex (ruptured central extension tendon)
- Mallet finger = flexion of DIP (avulsion)
- Dupuytren's contracture = flexion of 4th & 5th digits
- Ganglion cyst = defined mass on dorsum of hand
- Pill-rolling tremor = Parkinsonism
- Liver flap = asterixis = flapping tremor resulting from the inability to maintain wrist extension with the forearm supported in a flexed position

Palpation Pearls

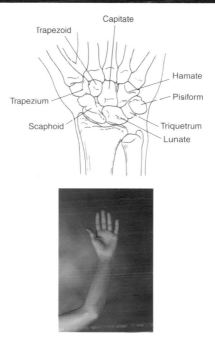

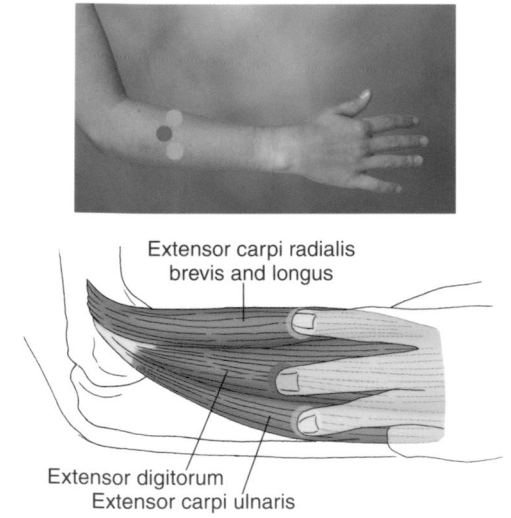

Extensor carpi radialis
brevis and longus

Extensor digitorum
Extensor carpi ulnaris

Wrist Flexor Muscles

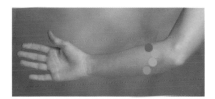

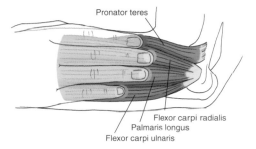

Pronator teres

Flexor carpi radialis

Palmaris longus

Flexor carpi ulnaris

Edema Assessment

Edema Assessment

Figure-8 Method to Assess Hand Edema (Palmar Surface)

1. Start distal to the lateral styloid process; go medial across the palm of the hand to the 5th MCP joint

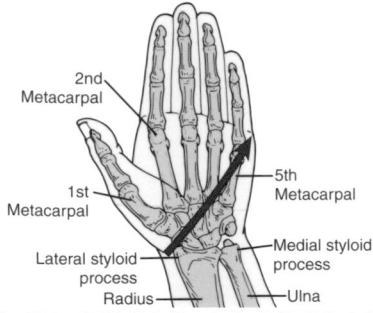

Source: Gulick, D. Sport Notes: Field & Clinical Examination Guide. FA Davis, Philadelphia, 2008, page 171.

2. Over the knuckles to the 2nd MCP joint

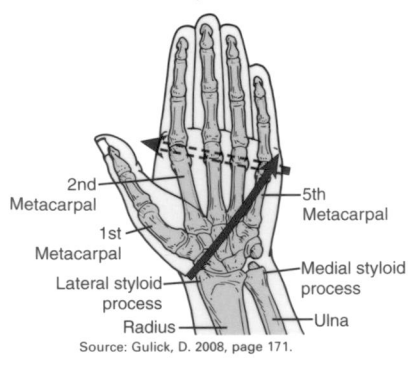

Source: Gulick, D. 2008, page 171.

3. Across the palm to the medial styloid process

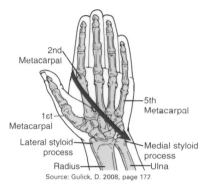

Source: Gulick, D. 2008, page 172.

4. Around the back of the wrist to the lateral styloid process

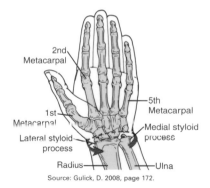

Source: Gulick, D. 2008, page 172.

Figure-8 Method to Assess Hand Edema (Dorsal Surface)

1. Start distal to the medial styloid process; go lateral across the back of the hand to the 2nd MCP joint

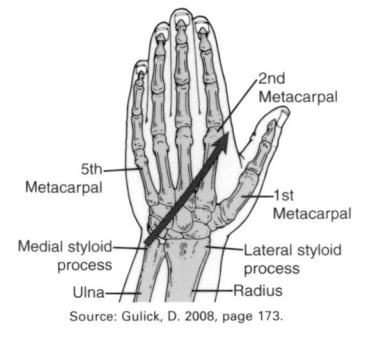

Source: Gulick, D. 2008, page 173.

2. Over the palmar aspect of the MCP joints to the 5th MCP joint

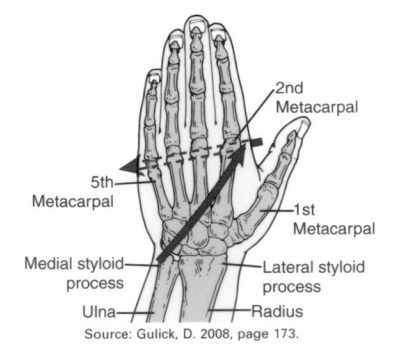

Source: Gulick, D. 2008, page 173.

3. Across the back of the hand to the lateral styloid process

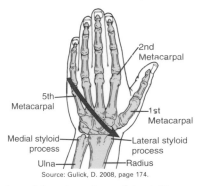

5th Metacarpal

2nd Metacarpal

1st Metacarpal

Medial styloid process

Lateral styloid process

Ulna

Radius

Source: Gulick, D. 2008, page 174.

4. Around the front of the wrist to the medial styloid process

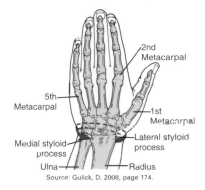

5th Metacarpal

2nd Metacarpal

1st Metacarpal

Medial styloid process

Lateral styloid process

Ulna

Radius

Source: Gulick, D. 2008, page 174.

2-Point Discrimination

Use a Disk-criminator to assess the minimal distance at which the client can distinguish the presence of 2 stimuli. The client should be able to distinguish 4 out of 5 or 7 out of 10 trials.

Grade	*Distance*
Normal	<6 mm
Fair	6–10 mm
Poor	11–15 mm

Semmes-Weinstein Monofilament Test

With client's eyes closed, clinician applies a perpendicular force to each test location beginning with the lowest monofilament. Record the number of the monofilament that the client feels before or just as the monofilament bends.

Test locations:

- Base of palm/wrist
- Between central palm & distal palm crease
- Between distal palm crease & web of finger
- Between web of finger & PIP joint
- Between PIP joint & DIP joint
- Between DIP joint & fingertip

Normal Values:

Monofilament #	*Result*
2.44–2.83	Normal sensation
3.22–4.56	Diminished light touch
4.74–6.10	Minimal light touch
6.10–6.65	Poor localization

Osteokinematics of the Wrist & Hand

Joint	Normal ROM	Normal End-feel(s)	Abnormal End-feel(s)
Radiocarpal	60°–80° flex 60°–70° ext 20°–30° RD/UD	Flex = firm/ligamentous/elastic Ext = firm/ligamentous/elastic RD = bony UD = firm/bony	Capsular = pronation & supination equally restricted
CMC thumb	70° abd 45°–50° flex	Elastic	Capsular = abd > ext
MCP 2–5	90° flex	Ext = elastic/capsular/ligamentous Flex = elastic/bony/firm/ligamentous Abd = firm/ligamentous	
MCP thumb	75°–90° flex	Flex = bony/firm/ligamentous/elastic Ext = firm/elastic	
IPs 2–5	100° PIP flex 80° DIP flex	PIP flex = firm/bony/elastic PIP ext = firm/ligamentous/elastic DIP flex = firm/ligamentous/elastic DIP ext = firm/ligamentous/elastic	

Radiocarpal	**Concave surface:** Radius & radioulnar disk	*To facilitate wrist flexion:* Proximal carpal rolls anterior & glides posterior on radius with distal carpal rolling anterior & gliding posterior on the proximal carpal	*To facilitate extension:* Proximal carpal rolls posterior & glides anterior & on radius with distal carpal rolling posterior & gliding anterior on the proximal carpal
	Convex surface: Proximal carpals	*To facilitate radial deviation:* Proximal carpal rolls lateral & glides medial on radius with distal carpal rolling lateral & gliding medial on the proximal carpal	*To facilitate ulnar deviation:* Proximal carpal rolls medial & glides lateral on radius with distal carpal rolling medial & gliding lateral on the proximal carpal
Distal radioulnar	**Concave surface:** Ulnar notch of radius **Convex surface:** Head of ulna	*To facilitate pronation:* Radius rolls & glides medially over the ulna	*To facilitate supination:* Radius rolls & glides laterally over the ulna

Continued

116

CMC thumb	Concave surface: Trapezii	*To facilitate thumb flexion:* Metacarpal rolls & glides medial on trapezium	*To facilitate thumb extension:* Metacarpal rolls & glides lateral on trapezium
CMC thumb	Convex surface: Metacarpal	*To facilitate thumb abduction:* Metacarpal rolls proximal & glides distal on trapezium	*To facilitate thumb adduction:* Metacarpal rolls distal & glides proximal on trapezium
MCP 2-5	Concave surface: Base of proximal phalanx	*To facilitate flexion:* Proximal phalanx rolls & glides anterior on metacarpal	*To facilitate extension:* Proximal phalanx rolls & glides posterior on metacarpal
MCP thumb	Convex surface: Head of metacarpal	*To facilitate thumb flexion:* Distal phalanx rolls & glides anterior on the proximal phalanx	*To facilitate thumb extension:* Distal phalanx rolls & glides posterior on the proximal phalanx
IP 2-5	Concave surface: Base of proximal phalanx Convex surface: Head of distal phalanx	*To facilitate flexion:* Distal phalanx rolls & glides anterior on the proximal phalanx	*To facilitate extension:* Distal phalanx rolls & glides posterior on the proximal phalanx

Strength & Function

Muscle Function

- Dorsal interossei = "divide" or separate fingers
- Palmar interossei & lumbricales = "pull" fingers together
- Flexor digitorum superficialis test = with finger in extension, isolate PIP flexion
- Flexor digitorum profundus test = with finger in extension, isolate DIP flexion
- Lumbrical test = flex MCP with IPs extended

- Power grips:
  - Cylindrical grip = FDP, FDS, FPL, FPB, OP, lumbricales, palmar interossei
  - Spherical grip = FDP, FDS, FPL, FPB, OP, lumbricales, dorsal interossei
  - Hook grip = FDS, FDP

Tools to Evaluate Grip Strength

- Hand-held dynamometer
- Jamar device—power grip in various positions
- Pinch meter:
  - Tip-to-tip = anterior interosseous nerve
  - Pad-to-pad = median nerve
  - 3-jaw chuck = ulnar nerve
- BP cuff inflated to 20 mm Hg; squeeze & assess pressure change

Objective Tests to Assess Hand Function

- Minnesota Rate of Manipulation Test
- Minnesota Manual Dexterity Test
- Purdue Pegboard Test
- Modified Moberg Pick-up Test

Quantitative Measure of Ulnar Impaction

- Assess grip in supinated & pronated wrist positions
- If grip ratio of supination:pronation is
  - = 1, there is no ulnar impaction
  - >1, ulnar impaction is present

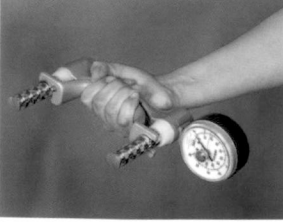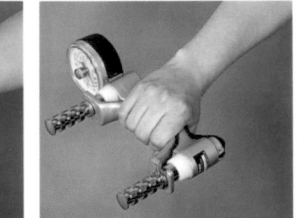

Brachial Plexus–Roots, Muscles, Deficits & Deformities

Nerve & Root	Muscles	Functional Deficits	Postural Deformity
Radial C5–8 T1	Anconeus, brachioradialis, ECRL, ECRB, extensor digitorum, APL, ECU, extensor indicis, extensor digiti minimi	■ Weak supination, wrist ext, finger flex, thumb abd ■ Weak grip due to loss of wrist stabilization	
Median C6–8 T1	Pronator teres, FCR, palmaris long, FDS, FPL, pronator quadratus, thenar eminence, lateral 2 lumbricales	■ Weak pronation, wrist flex & RD ■ Weak thumb flex & abd ■ Weak grip & pinch ■ Ape hand	
Ulnar C7–8 T1	FCU, palmaris brevis, hypothenar eminence, adductor pollicis, medial 2 lumbricales, interossei	■ Weak wrist flex & UD ■ Weak 5th finger flex ■ Weak finger abd/add ■ Benediction sign (Bishop's deformity)	Claw hand = median & ulnar

Source for top figure: From Levangie, PK, & Norkin, CC. Joint Structure & Function: A Comprehensive Analysis. 3rd ed. FA Davis, Philadelphia, 2001, page 107.

Neural Tissue Provocation Tests

■ See Alerts/Alarms page 14.

Wrist & Hand Tests

CLAMP SIGN

Purpose: Assess for scaphoid fx
Position: Wrist in pronation & extension
Technique: Grasp web space of the thumb between clinician's thumb & index finger & gently stress the wrist into UD
Interpretation: + test = pain in the anatomical snuff box
Statistics: Sensitivity = 52% & specificity = 100%

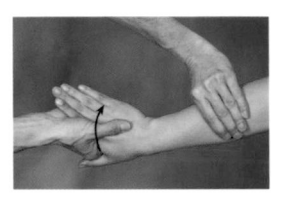

WATSON'S TEST (Scaphoid shift maneuver)

Purpose: Assess for scaphoid instability
Position: Supinated in neutral
Technique: From the radial side, the clinician uses his thumb on the palmar side & index finger on dorsal side to apply pressure to the distal scaphoid while moving the wrist from UD to RD
Interpretation: + test = removal of pressure will produce a palpable click & dorsal wrist pain

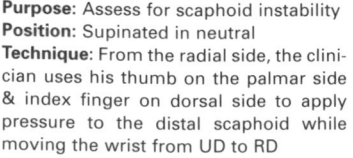

FINKELSTEIN'S TEST

Purpose: Assess for de Quervain's syndrome
Position: Form a fist around the thumb
Technique: Ulnarly deviate the wrist
Interpretation: + test = pain along EPB & APL

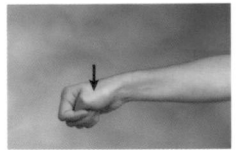

WRIST VARUS TEST

Purpose: Assess RCL
Position: Stabilize radius/ulna proximal to wrist in neutral position
Technique: Apply a varus stress to the wrist
Interpretation: + test = joint line pain or gapping/instability

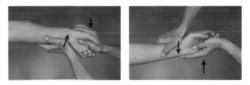

Source: Gulick, D., 2008, page 125.

WRIST VALGUS TEST

Purpose: Assess UCL
Position: Stabilize radius/ulna proximal to wrist in neutral position
Technique: Apply a valgus stress to the wrist
Interpretation: + test = joint line pain or gapping/instability

PHALANX VARUS/VALGUS TEST

Purpose: Assess MCL & LCL
Position: With finger(s) in neutral, stabilize the proximal phalanx
Technique: Apply a varus/valgus stress via the distal phalanx
Interpretation: + test = joint line pain or gapping/instability

PHALEN'S TEST

Purpose: Assess for CTS
Position: Hands relaxed
Technique: Maximally flex the wrists so the dorsal surfaces of the hands are in full contact with each other; hold for up to 1 minute
Interpretation: + test = numbness or tingling into the median nerve distribution
Statistics: Sensitivity = 34%–93% & specificity = 48%–93%

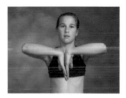

REVERSE PHALEN'S TEST (Prayer Sign)

Purpose: Assess for CTS

Position: Hands relaxed

Technique: Maximally extend the wrists so the palms of the hands are in full contact with each other; hold for up to 1 minute

Interpretation: + test = numbness or tingling into the median nerve distribution

Statistics: Sensitivity = 88% & specificity = 93%

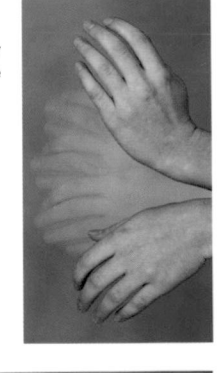

FLICK MANEUVER

Purpose: Assess for CTS

Position: Hands relaxed

Technique: Vigorously shake the hands repeatedly

Interpretation: + test = paresthesia into the median nerve distribution

Statistics: Sensitivity = 37% & specificity = 74%

TINEL'S SIGN

Purpose: Assess for CTS

Position: UE supported in supination

Technique: Tap the volar surface of the wrist

Interpretation: + test = tingling into the median nerve distribution

Statistics: CTS: Sensitivity = 27%–79% & specificity = 65%–98%

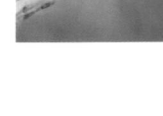

Wrist tests	Sensitivity	Specificity
• Flick + Phalen's	49	62
• Flick + Tinel's	46	68
• Phalen's + Tinel's	41	72

FROMENT'S SIGN

Purpose: Assess for adductor pollicis weakness 2° ulnar nerve paralysis
Position: Client holds a paper between thumb & index finger
Technique: Clinician tries to tug the paper away
Interpretation: + test = flexion of thumb DIP via FPL will result if the adductor pollicis muscle is impaired by an ulnar nerve px

WARTENBERG'S TEST

Purpose: Assess ulnar nerve for entrapment at the elbow
Position: UE relaxed in a supported position
Technique: Resist 5th digit adduction
Interpretation: + test = weakness of the 5th digit adduction

MURPHY'S SIGN

Purpose: Assess for lunate dislocation
Position: Make a fist
Technique: Observe alignment of MC joints
Interpretation: + test = 3rd MCP is level with 2nd & 4th, (normally 3rd MCP should project beyond 2nd & 4th)

ALLEN'S TEST

Purpose: Test for occlusion of radial or ulnar artery
Position: Hand relaxed, supported in supination
Technique: Clinician compresses both radial & ulnar arteries at the wrist while client clenches hand several times to drain blood out. With client's hand open, clinician releases pressure on the radial artery—normal hand coloration should return in <5 seconds. Repeat & release ulnar artery

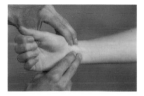

Interpretation: + test = difference between the 2 vessels with respect to refill time or taking >5 seconds for coloration of tissue to return to normal

TFCC LOAD TEST

Purpose: Assess TFCC
Position: Wrist in ulnar deviation
Technique: Apply a longitudinal load through the 5th metacarpal bone to the TFCC
Interpretation: + test = pain @ TFCC
Statistics: Sensitivity = 100%

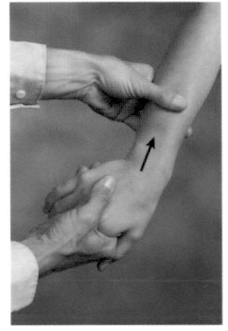

TFCC PRESS TEST/ SUPINATED LIFT TEST

Purpose: Assess TFCC
Position: Elbow flexed at 90° & forearm supinated
Technique: Client is asked to lift up against resistance (like lifting a table via wrist flexion)
Interpretation: + test = compression with UD will ↑ pain @ TFCC
Statistics: Sensitivity = 100%

Pathology/Mechanism	Signs/Symptoms
Colles' or Smith's Fracture—distal radial fractures 2° FOOSH with extreme wrist extension; common in adults >50 yo, whereas children = greenstick or epiphyseal growth plate	■ TTP in anatomical snuffbox ■ Edema & ecchymosis ■ Structural deformity with limited ROM ■ Confirmed via PA, oblique & lateral x-rays (Colles' fx = distal fragment angles dorsal & Smith's fx = distal fragment angles palmar)
Dupuytren's Contracture—flexion contracture with thickening of palmar fascia of 4th & 5th digits; etiology is unknown (if associated with DM, may involved 3rd & 4th digits), epilepsy, & (+) family hx; most common in ♂ >40 yo	■ Nodule in the palmar aponeurosis of the ulnar side & tightening of the natatory ligament ■ Usually no pain but MCPs are unable to extend ■ May reappear again weeks or years later ■ Confirmed with CT or MRI
Trigger Finger—results when the demand for manual dexterity & fist clenching tasks exceed the lubricating capacity of the synovial fluid; ↑ incidence in DM & people >40 yo	■ Tender nodules in flexor tendon @ MC head that moves with the tendon ■ No active finger flexion ■ Finger locks in flexion in AM; extension only can be performed passively & there is slight pain with clicking/grating when passively moved ■ Diagnosis confirmed with CT or MRI
De Quervain's Syndrome—tenosynovitis of the abductor pollicis longus & extensor pollicis brevis > extensor pollicis longus; insidious onset related to pinching or grasping tasks	■ No numbness, tingling, or edema ■ AROM of thumb is painful ■ Pain radiates into distal radial forearm ■ Pulses are normal ■ (+) Finkelstein's test ■ Confirmed with CT or MRI; should r/o gout

Continued

Pathology/Mechanism	Signs/Symptoms
Carpal Tunnel Syndrome (CTS)—an overuse injury related to repetitive trauma; occurs in ♀ > ♂; may occur during pregnancy	■ Thenar atrophy but no swelling or trophic changes ■ Night-time numbness of hand (median nerve pattern) ■ Thumb weakness & loss of opposition/abduction—specifically APB (beware of substitution of APL, innervated by the radial nerve) ■ (+) Tests: Phalen's, Reverse Phalen's, Flick, Neural provocation, & Tinel sign; (–) TOS ■ Normal pulses (radial & ulnar arteries do not pass through tunnel) ■ Sensation of palm is spared ■ Need to r/o C-spine problem ■ Confirmed with CT or MRI
Pronator Syndrome—compression of the median nerve via pronator muscle	■ Client c/o "heaviness" in the UE ■ Pain with overpressure into pronation (median nerve distribution) ■ (-) Phalen's & Tinel's sign, ↓ NCV ■ TTP over pronator teres (~4 cm distal to cubital crease) ■ Mimics CTS but there is no night pain or weakness ■ Confirmed with MRI or CT
Gamekeeper's Thumb—ulnar collateral ligament injury 2° a forceful radial deviation of the thumb	■ Localized pain & swelling ■ TTP @ UCL ■ (+) Valgus stress ■ Confirmed with MRI, need to r/o fx & avulsion
Triangular Fibro Cartilage Complex (TFCC)—injury is the result of forceful rotation of forearm or FOOSH in pronation	■ (+) Tests: Load & Press test ■ >1 grip ratio of supination:pronation ■ TTP @ TFCC ■ Confirmed with MRI or arthrogram
Ganglion Cyst—most common mass in the wrist, etiology unknown, may be associated with repetitive motions	■ Defined round mass in the wrist ■ May be painful with motion or compression ■ Not revealed on x-ray, MRI, CT

Continued

Pathology/Mechanism	Signs/Symptoms
Lunate Dislocation—results from FOOSH	■ (+) Murphy's sign ■ TTP @ lunate with localized swelling ■ Painful wrist ROM ■ May cause paresthesia if median nerve is involved ■ Confirmed with x-ray, need to r/o fx

Tendon Rupture—results from trauma	■ Edema & TTP are tendon specific
	■ Failure to actively move a joint:
	  ■ EPL = no thumb IP ext (mallet finger)
	  ■ FPL = no thumb IP flex
	  ■ ED = no isolated long finger ext (mallet finger)
	  ■ FDP = no DIP flexion (jersey finger)
	  ■ FS = no PIP flexion
	■ Confirmed with MRI or CT; need to r/o fx or avulsion

Raynaud's Syndrome—cold-induced reflex digital vasoconstriction & ischemia	■ Pallor, cyanosis then redness of digits (cyclic) ■ (–) TOS test(s) ■ Clear C-spine ■ ROM, strength, & sensation = WNL ■ Confirmed via Doppler
Complex Regional Pain Syndrome—etiology unknown, may occur after trauma See stages next page.	■ Hyperalgesia & hyperhydrosis ■ Capsular tightness & stiffness ■ Muscle atrophy & osteoporosis ■ Trophic changes & edema ■ Vasomotor instability

Complex Regional Pain Syndrome

Stage 1	• Burning, aching, tenderness, joint stiffness • Swelling, temperature changes • ↑ nail growth & ↑ hair on hands
Stage 2	• ↑ Pain, swelling, joint stiffness • Pain becomes less localized • Change in skin color & texture
Stage 3	• Pain radiates all the way up the arm • ↓ NCV • Muscle atrophy

Ligaments of the neck

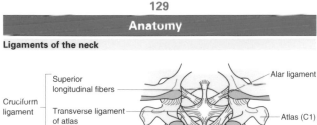

Muscles of the neck & face (lateral view)

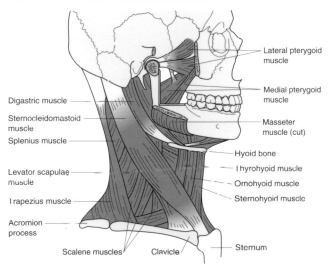

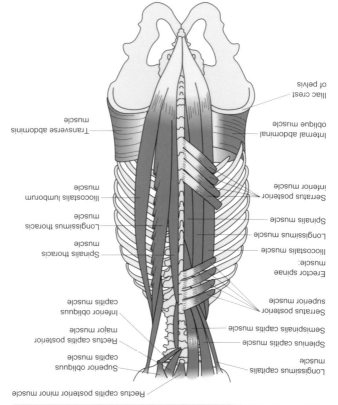

Deep muscles of the neck & back

Superficial muscles of the neck & back

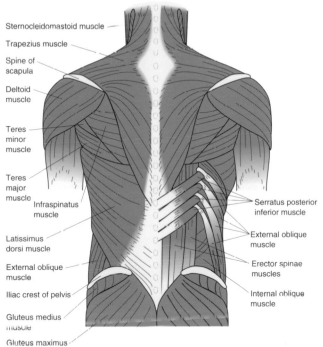

Sternocleidomastoid muscle

Trapezius muscle

Spine of scapula

Deltoid muscle

Teres minor muscle

Teres major muscle

Infraspinatus muscle

Latissimus dorsi muscle

External oblique muscle

Iliac crest of pelvis

Gluteus medius muscle

Gluteus maximus muscle

Serratus posterior inferior muscle

External oblique muscle

Erector spinae muscles

Internal oblique muscle

Abdominal muscles

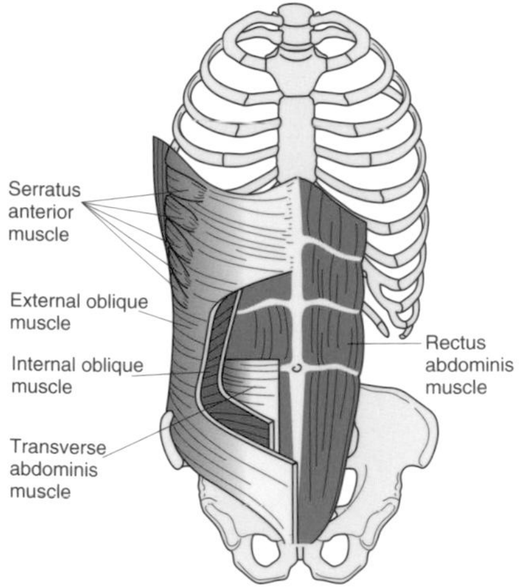

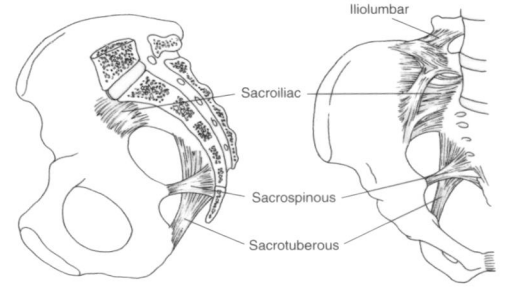

Serratus anterior muscle

External oblique muscle

Internal oblique muscle

Transverse abdominis muscle

Rectus abdominis muscle

Ligaments of the pelvis

Iliolumbar

Sacroiliac

Sacrospinous

Sacrotuberous

Source: From Cailliet, R. Low Back Pain Syndrome, 3rd ed. FA Davis, Philadelphia, 1983, page 196.

Spine Medical Red Flags

- Individuals <20 & >55 yo with persistent night pain, change in B&B control, (B) LE signs, PMH of CA, nonmechanical pain, SED rate >25
- Mid-thoracic pain = MI, GB
- Pain from 6th–10th thoracic vertebra = peptic ulcer
- History of prostate CA
- Pulsing LBP = vascular problem (aortic aneurysm)
- Faun's beard = spina bifida
- Café au lait spots = neurofibromatosis
- Upper back/neck pain that ↑ with deep breathing, coughing, laughing & ↓ with breath holding; recent hx may include fever URI, flu, MI = pericarditis
- Enlarged cervical lymph nodes, severe pruritus, irregular fever = Hodgkin's disease
- Pain at McBurney's point = ⅓–½ the distance from (R) ASIS to umbilicus; tenderness = appendicitis

Risk Factors for Chronicity of Spinal Dysfunction

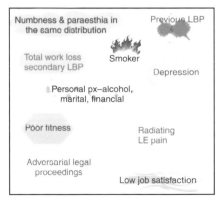

Numbness & paraesthia in the same distribution

Previous LBP

Total work loss secondary LBP

Smoker

Depression

Personal px–alcohol, marital, financial

Poor fitness

Radiating LE pain

Adversarial legal proceedings

Low job satisfaction

Neck Disability Index For Chronic Pain

Pain Intensity
__ I have no pain at the moment
__ The pain is very mild at the moment
__ The pain is moderate at the moment
__ The pain is fairly severe at the moment
__ The pain is very severe at the moment
__ The pain is the worst imaginable at the moment

Work
__ I can do as much as I want to
__ I can only do my usual work but not more
__ I can do most of my usual work, but not more
__ I cannot do my usual work
__ I can hardly do any usual work at all
__ I can't do any work at all

Personal Care (washing, dressing, etc.)
__ I can look after myself normally w/o causing extra pain
__ I can look after myself normally but it causes extra pain
__ It is painful to look after myself & I am slow & careful
__ I need some help but manage most of my personal care
__ I need help every day in most aspect of self care
__ I cannot get dressed, wash with difficulty & stay in Bed

Concentration
__ I can concentrate fully when I want to with no difficulty
__ I can concentrate fully when I want to with slight difficulty
__ I have a fair degree of difficulty concentrating when I want
__ I have a lot of difficulty concentrating when I want
__ I have a great deal of difficulty concentrating when I want
__ I cannot concentrate at all

Lifting
__ I can lift heavy weights without extra pain
__ I can lift heavy weights but it gives extra pain
__ Pain prevents me from lifting heavy weights off the floor, but I can manage if they are on a table
__ Pain prevents me from lifting heavy weights but I can manage if they are conveniently placed
__ I can lift only very light weights
__ I cannot lift or carry anything at all

Driving
__ I can drive my car without neck pain
__ I can drive my car as long as I want with slight neck pain
__ I can drive my car as long as I want with moderate neck pain
__ I can't drive my car as long as I want because of moderate neck pain
__ I can hardly drive at all because of severe neck pain
__ I can't drive my car at all

Continued

Neck Disability Index For Chronic Pain—*cont'd*

Reading
- __ I can read as much as I want with no pain in my neck
- __ I can read as much as I want with slight pain in my neck
- __ I can read as much as I want with moderate pain in my neck
- __ I can't read as much as I want because of moderate pain in my neck
- __ I can hardly read at all because of severe pain in my neck
- __ I cannot read at all

Recreation
- __ I am able to engage in all my recreational activities with no neck pain
- __ I am able to engage in all my recreational activities with some neck pain
- __ I am able to engage in most but not all of my usual recreational activities because of neck pain
- __ I am able to engage in a few of my usual recreational activities with some neck pain
- __ I can hardly do any recreational activities because of neck pain
- __ I can't do any recreational activities at all

Headache
- __ I have no headaches at all
- __ I have slight headaches which come infrequently
- __ I have moderate headaches which come infrequently
- __ I have moderate headaches which come frequently
- __ I have severe headaches which come infrequently
- __ I have headaches almost all the time

Sleeping
- __ I have no trouble sleeping My sleep is slightly disturbed (<1-hr sleep loss)
- __ My sleep is mildly disturbed (1- to 2-hr sleep loss)
- __ My sleep is moderately disturbed (2- to 3-hr sleep loss)
- __ My sleep is greatly disturbed (3- to 5-hr sleep loss)
- __ My sleep is completely disturbed (5- to 7-hr sleep loss)

Score:

Scoring: The items are scored in descending order with the top statement = 0 & the bottom statement = 5. All subsections are added together for a cumulative score. The higher the score, the greater the disability.

Source: From the Journal of Manipulation and Physiological Therapeutics. 14(7):561–570, 1991.

Oswestry Low Back Pain Questionnaire

In every section, please mark the one response that most closely describes your problem:

Pain Intensity

__ I can tolerate the pain without using pain killers

__ The pain is bad but I manage without pain killers

__ Pain killers give complete relief from pain

__ Pain killers give moderate relief from pain

__ Pain killers give very little relief from pain

__ Pain killers have no effect on the pain; I don't use them

Personal Care (washing, dressing, etc.)

__ I can look after myself normally without causing extra pain

__ I can look after myself normally but it causes extra pain

__ It is painful to look after myself & I am slow & careful

__ I need some help but manage most of my personal care

__ I need help every day in most aspect of self care

__ I cannot get dressed, wash with difficulty & stay in bed

Standing

__ I can stand as long as I want without extra pain

__ I can stand as long as I want but it given me extra pain

__ Pain prevents me from standing for >1 hour

__ Pain prevents me from standing >½ hour

__ Pain prevents me from standing >10 minutes

__ Pain prevents me from standing at all

Sleeping

__ Pain does not prevent me from sleeping well

__ I can sleep well only by using tablets

__ Even when I take tablets, I have <6 hours sleep

__ Even when I take tablets, I have <4 hours sleep

__ Even when I take tablets, I have <2 hours sleep

__ Pain prevents me from sleeping at all

Continued

Oswestry Low Back Pain Questionnaire—cont'd

Lifting

___ I can lift heavy weights without extra pain
___ I can lift heavy weights but it gives extra pain
___ Pain prevents me from lifting heavy weights off the floor, but I can manage if they are on a table
___ Pain prevents me from lifting heavy weights but I can manage if they are conveniently placed
___ I can lift only very light weights
___ I cannot lift or carry anything at all

Walking

___ Pain does not prevent me walking any distances
___ Pain prevents me walking more than 1 mile
___ Pain prevents me walking more than ½ mile
___ Pain prevents me walking more than ¼ mile
___ I can only walk using a stick or crutches
___ I am in bed most of the time & have to crawl to the toilet

Sex Life

___ My sex life is normal & causes no extra pain
___ My sex life is normal but causes some extra pain
___ My sex life is nearly normal but is very painful
___ My sex life is severely restricted by pain
___ My sex life is nearly absent because of pain
___ Pain prevents any sex life at all

Social Life

___ My social life is normal & gives me no extra pain
___ My social life is normal but increases the degree of pain
___ Pain has no significant effect on my social life apart from limiting my more energetic interests (e.g., dancing)
___ Pain has restricted my social life & I do not go out as often
___ Pain has restricted my social life to my home
___ I have no social life because of pain

Oswestry Low Back Pain Questionnaire—*cont'd*

Sitting

___ I can sit in any chair as long as I like
___ I can only sit in my favorite chair as long as I like
___ Pain prevents me sitting more than 1 hour
___ Pain prevents me sitting more than ½ hour
___ Pain prevents me sitting more than 10 minutes
___ Pain prevents me sitting at all

Traveling

___ I can travel anywhere without extra pain
___ I can travel anywhere but it gives me extra pain
___ Pain is bad but I manage journeys over 2 hours
___ Pain restricts me to journeys < 1 hour
___ Pain restricts me to short necessary journeys under 30 minutes
___ Pain prevents me from traveling except to the doctor or hospital

Score:

Scoring: The items are scored in descending order with the top statement = 0 & the bottom statement = 5. The sum of the score is multiplied by 2.

Results: 0–20% = minimal disability; 20%–40% = moderate disability; 40%–60% = severe disability; 60%–80% = crippled; 80%–100% = bed bound or symptom magnification

Source: From Physiotherapy, 66(8):271–273, 1980.

Ransford Pain Drawings

Indicate where your pain is located & what type of pain you feel at the present time. Use the symbols below to describe your pain. Do not indicate areas of pain which are not related to your present injury or condition.

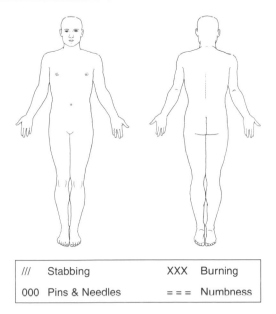

///	Stabbing	XXX	Burning
000	Pins & Needles	= = =	Numbness

Ransford Scoring System

- Unreal drawings (score 2 points for any of the following)
  - Total leg pain
  - Front of leg pain
  - Anterior tibial pain
  - Back of leg & knee pain
  - Circumferential thigh pain
  - Lateral whole leg pain
  - Bilateral foot pain
  - Circumferential foot pain
  - Anterior knee & ankle pain
  - Scattered pain throughout while leg
  - Entire abdomen pain
- Drawings with "expansion" or "magnification" of pain (1–2 points)
  - Back pain radiating into iliac crest, groin, & anterior perineum
  - Pain drawn outside of diagram
- Additional explanations, circles, lines, arrows (1 point each)
- Painful areas drawn in (score 1 for small areas & 2 for large areas)

Interpretation: A score of 3 or more points is thought to represent a pain perception that may be influenced by psychological factors

Score:

Short Form McGill Pain Questionnaire

Instructions: Read the following descriptions of pain and mark the number which indicates the level of pain you feel in each category according to the following scale:

	1 = None	2 = Mild	3 = Moderate	4 = Severe
Throbbing				
Shooting				
Stabbing				
Sharp				
Cramping				
Gnawing				
Hot-Burning				
Aching				
Heavy				
Tender				
Splitting				
Tiring-Exhausting				
Sickening				
Fearful				
Punishing-Cruel				

Total Score: _____
The higher the score, the more intense the pain.

Present Pain Intensity Index

Instructions: Use the descriptors below to indicate your current level of pain

0 = No Pain
1 = Mild
2 = Discomforting
3 = Distressing
4 = Horrible
5 = Excruciating

Cutaneous Pain Referral Patterns from the Viscera

Viscera	Segmental Level	Referral Pattern
Pharynx		Ipsilateral ear
Heart	T1–5	Sternum, neck
Bronchi-lungs	T2–4	Shoulder, pect, arm L>R
Esophagus	T5–6	Neck, arms, sternum (level of the nipple)
Gastric	T6–10	Lower thoracic to upper abdomen
GB	T7–9	Upper abdomen (epigastric area), lower scapula, T/L
Pancreas	T8–9	Upper lumbar, upper abdomen
Kidneys	T10–L1	Upper lumbar, umbilical area
Bladder	T11–12	Lower abdomen, lower lumbar, groin

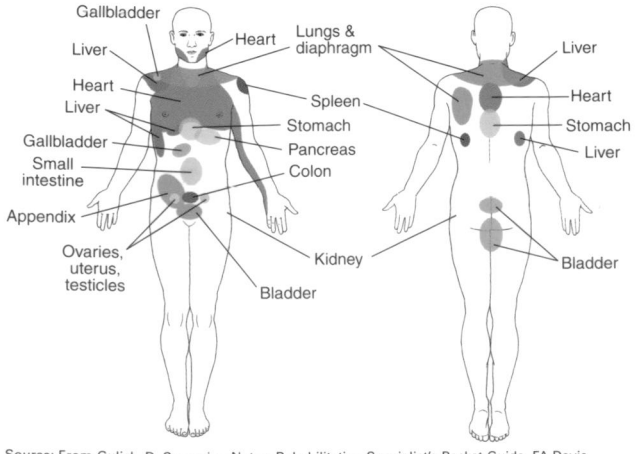

Source: From Gulick, D. Screening Notes: Rehabilitation Specialist's Pocket Guide. FA Davis, Philadelphia, 2006, page 11.

Headaches

Type of Pain	Possible Etiology
Acute	Trauma, infection, impending CVA
Chronic	Eye strain, ETOH, inadequate ventilation
Severe & intense	Meningitis, aneurysm, brain tumor
Throbbing/pulsating	Migraine, fever, hypertension, aortic insufficiency
Constant	Muscle contraction/guarding
AM pain	Sinusitis (with discharge), ETOH, hypertension, sleeping position
Afternoon pain	Eye strain, muscle tension
Night	Intracranial disease, nephritis
Forehead	Sinusitis, nephritis
Temporal	Eye or ear px, migraine
Occipital	Herniated disk, eye strain, hypertension
Parietal	Meningitis, constipation, tumor
Face	Sinusitis, trigeminal neuralgia, dental px, tumor
Stabbing pain	With ear fullness, tinnitus, vertigo = otitis media
Severe pain	With fever, (+) Kernig's sign = meningitis
Severe, sudden pain	With ↑ BP = subarachnoid hemorrhage
Intermittent pain	With fluctuating consciousness = subdural hematoma

Dermatomes

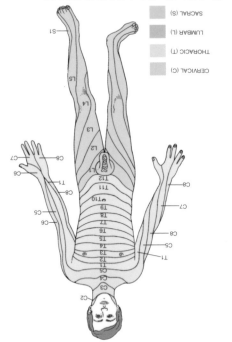

CERVICAL (C)

THORACIC (T)

LUMBAR (L)

SACRAL (S)

Source: From Taber's 20th edition, FA Davis, Philadelphia, 2005, p. 571.

144

Muscle Pain Referral Patterns

Scalenes

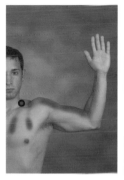

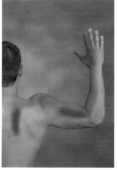

Sternocleidomastoid

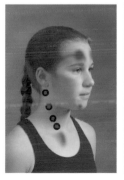

Trapezius

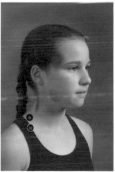

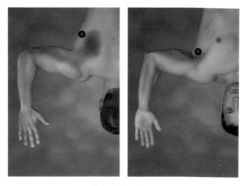

Gluteus maximus

Quadratus Lumborum

Latissimus dorsi

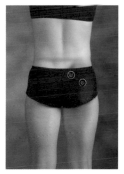

Palpation Pearls

Landmarks

Vertebral Level	Identification Strategy
C1	1 fingerwidth below mastoid process 2 fingerwidths below occipital protuberance
C2	Angle of the mandible 3 fingerwidths below occipital protuberance
C3–4	Posterior to hyoid bone
C7	Base of neck (prominent posterior spinous process)
T2	Superior angle of scapula & jugular notch
T7	Inferior angle of the scapula
T10	Xiphoid process
T12	12th rib
L3	Posterior to umbilicus
L4	Iliac crest
S2	Level of PSIS
Tip of coccyx	Ischial tuberosities

- **Anterior neck muscles** (medial & anterior to lateral & posterior) = sternal branch of SCM, sternohyoid, clavicular branch of SCM, subclavian vein, anterior scalene, subclavian artery, brachial plexus, middle scalene, posterior scalene, levator scapula
- **Posterior neck muscles** (medial to lateral) = rectus capitis, semispinalis, splenius capitis, longissimus capitis
- **Posterior thoracic & lumbar spine** (medial to lateral) = spinalis, longissimus, iliocostalis

Pathology & Compensatory Strategies That Influence Limb Length

Lengthen of LE	Shortening of LE
■ Anterior rotation of SI	■ Posterior rotation of SI
■ Extension of hip	■ Hike/flex hip; IR of hip
■ ER of hip	■ Circumduct LE
■ Supination of foot	■ Flexion of the knee
	■ Varus/valgus of knee
	■ Pronation of foot

ROM

Cervical Normal Ranges

Motion	Segment(s)	Degrees
FB/BB	Suboccipital (nod)	20°–25°
	Mid-cervical	30°–35°
SB	Suboccipital (primarily A/A)	20°
	Mid-cervical	25°
Rot	Suboccipital	35°
	Mid-cervical	45°

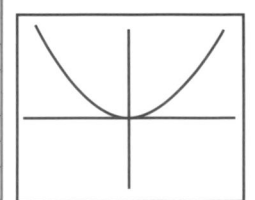

Thoracic Normal Ranges

Motion	Degrees
FB	20°–40°
BB	15°–30°
SB	25°–30°
Rot	5°–20°

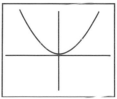

Lumbar Normal Ranges

Motion	Degrees
FB = greatest @ L4–5	40°–60°
BB	20°–25°
SB = greatest @ L3–4	15°–35°
Rot = greatest @ L4–S1	5°–20°

Assessment Methods for Lumbar ROM:

- **Schober's Test** = find L4 & mark 5 cm above & 10 cm below. Have client FB & measure distance between 2 points; Normal > 5 cm increase
- **Modified Schober's Test** = initial landmark is a mark between the PSIS & then marks at 5 & 10 cm above. Measure the distance between the points to reflect the amount of flexion at each lumbar region
- **Inclinometer** – (BROM) in standing – place 1 inclinometer on the sacrum & 1 inclinometer over T12 spinous process. Have client FB & the amount of lumbar flexion is calculated by subtracting the sacral angles from the T12 angles

Basic Principles
- Hip motion is coupled with innominate motion
- Lumbar motion is coupled with sacral motion
- Nutation means "to nod" = anterior tilt in sagittal plane
- Counternutation = posterior tilt in sagittal plane

Joint motion	Innominate	Sacrum
Hip flexion	Ipsilateral posterior rotation	∅
Hip extension	Ipsilateral anterior rotation	∅
Hip IR	Ipsilateral IR or Inflare	∅
Hip ER	Ipsilateral ER or Outflare	∅
Lumbar FB	Anterior rotation	Nutation then counternutation
Lumbar BB	Slight posterior rotation	Nutation
Lumbar rotation	Ipsilateral posterior rotation & contralateral anterior rotation	Nutates ipsilaterally
Lumbar SB	Ipsilateral anterior rotation & contralateral posterior rotation	Ipsilateral SB ipsilateral & contralateral SB contralateral

Atlanto-occipital joint	Concave surface: Superior atlas facet Convex surface: Occiput	To facilitate FB: Occiput rolls anterior & glides posterior	To facilitate BB: Occiput rolls posterior & glides anterior
Atlantoaxial joint	Concave surface: Inferior atlas facet Convex surface: Superior axis facet	To facilitate rotation: Atlas pivots on axis	To facilitate rotation: Atlas pivots on axis
*Intracervical segments	Facets are oriented @ 45° in horizontal & frontal planes	To facilitate FB: Inferior facet of superior vertebrae glides up & FW on superior facet of inferior vertebrae	To facilitate BB: Inferior facet of superior vertebrae glides down & back on superior facet of inferior vertebrae
		To facilitate rotation: Inferior facet of superior vertebra glides posterior & inferior on ipsilateral side & anterior & superior on contralateral side	To facilitate SR: Inferior facet of superior vertebra glides inferior & posterior & on ipsilateral side & superior & anterior on contralateral side
*Intracervical segments	Facets are oriented @ 45° in horizontal & frontal planes	To facilitate protraction: Craniocervical segments extend while mid-low cervical segments flex	To facilitate retraction: Craniocervical segments flex while mid-low cervical segments extend

Continued

**Thoracic & Lumbar	Thoracic facets are oriented in the frontal plane	To facilitate flexion: Inferior facet of superior vertebra glides up & FW on superior facet of inferior vertebra	To facilitate extension: Inferior facet of superior vertebra glides down & BW on superior facet of inferior vertebra
	Lumbar facets are oriented in the saggital plane		
		To facilitate rotation: Inferior facet of contralateral superior vertebra compresses against superior facet of inferior facet & inferior facet of ipsilateral superior vertebra separates from superior facet of inferior vertebra	To facilitate SB: Inferior facet of superior vertebra slides up on the contralateral side of SB & down on the ipsilateral side of the SB motion

*Left SB & left rotation are coupled motions in the cervical spine.

**Right rotation & left SB are coupled motions in the lumbar spine.

Posture

Cervical

- ↑ FH = ↑ compression forces on anterior, lower c-vertebra & posterior facets; levator scapula can help to resist these stresses but may result in MTrP or adaptive shortening
- Shoulder protraction may result from GH or AC instability

Swayback (↑ kyphosis & ↓ lordosis)

- Alters the resting position of the scapula & alters the GH rhythm
- Tight hip extensors
- Weak hip flexors or lower abdominals
- Generalized ↓ strength
- Genu recurvatum = ↑ stress on posterior knee & compression of anterior knee
- Posterior pelvic tilt
- ↑ stress/elongation of anterior hip joint & posterior t-spine
- Shortening of posterior hip ligaments & anterior t-spine ligaments
- Forward head & shoulders

Lordosis

- Tight hip flexors or back extensors
- Weak hip extensors or abdominals
- Anterior pelvic tilt
- ↑ shear forces on lumbar vertebra
- ↑ compression forces on lumbar facets
- Stress & elongation of anterior spinal ligaments
- Narrowing of L-intervertebral foramen

Flatback (↓ kyphosis & ↓ lordosis)

- Forward head, posterior pelvic tilt, knee flexion
- Tight hip extensors
- Weak hip flexors & back extensors
- Compressive forces in posterior hip jt, anterior L-spine & posterior T-spine

Neuromuscular Relationships

Motion Segment	Nerve Root	Myotome	Dermatome	Reflex
Occ–C1	C1	∅	Skull vertex	∅
C1–2	C2	Neck flexion—Rectus capitis & SCM	Temple, forehead, occiput	∅
C2–3	C3	Neck SB—Trapezius & Splenius capitis	Cheek, neck	∅
C3–4	C4	Shoulder elevation—Levator scapula & Trapezius	Clavicle & upper scapula	∅
C4–5	C5	Shoulder abd—Deltoid, Supra/i nfraspinatus, Biceps	Anterior arm—shoulder to base of 1st digit	Biceps
C5–6	C6	Elbow flex/Wrist ext—Biceps, ECRL, ECRB, Supinator	Anterior arm to lateral forearm, 1st & 2nd digit	Brachioradialis
C6–7	C7	Elbow ext/Wrist flex—Triceps, FCU, FCR	Lateral forearm, 2nd, 3rd, & 4th digits	Triceps
C7–T1	C8	Thumb ext/UD—EPL, EPB, FCU, ECU	Medial arm & forearm to 4th & 5th digits	Triceps
T1–2	T1	∅	Medial forearm to base of 5th digit	∅
T2–3	T2	∅	Pectoralis & mid-scapula to medial upper arm & elbow	∅

Continued

Motion Segment	Nerve Root	Myotome	Dermatome	Reflex
T3–5	T3–5	∅	Upper thorax	∅
T5–7	T5–7	∅	Costal margins	∅
T8–12	T8–12	∅	Abdominal & lumbar regions	∅
T12–L1	I 1	Iliacus	Back to trochanter & inguinal region	∅
L1–2	L2	Psoas, iliacus, & adductors	Back to mid-anterior thigh to knee	Cremasteric
L2–3	L3	Quads	Back & upper buttock to distal anterior thigh & knee	Adductor
L3–4	L4	Anterior tibialis	Medial buttock to lateral thigh, medial tibia & big toe	Patella
L4–5	L5	Extensor hallucis longus	Posterior lateral thigh, lateral leg, dorsum of foot, & toes 1, 2, 3	Tib posterior, Med hamstrings
L5–S2	S1–2	Gluteals, hamstrings, peroneals, gastroc-soleus	Posterior thigh & leg, lateral foot & heel	Achilles
S2–3	S3	∅	Groin, medial thigh to knee	∅
S3–4	S4	Bladder & rectum	Perineum & genitals	∅

SLUMP TEST

Purpose: Assess neural mobility

Position: Sitting with trunk in slumped posture

Technique: While sustaining neck flexion, sequentially add knee extension of 1 LE & then dorsiflexion; repeat with other LE

Interpretation: + test = reproduction of symptoms; compare bilaterally

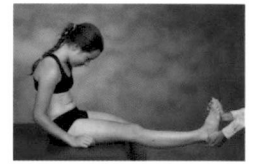

Statistics: Sensitivity = 83% & specificity = 55%

SPURLING'S TEST/ CERVICAL QUADRANT SIGN

Purpose: Assess nerve roots & IVF

Position: Seated

Technique: Stand behind client with clinician's fingers interlocked on top of head & compress (axial load) with c-spine in slight extension & lateral flexion

Interpretation: + test = referred or reproduction of pain; implicates a variety of structures related to compromise of the IVF

Statistics: Sensitivity = 30%–60% & specificity = 74%–100%

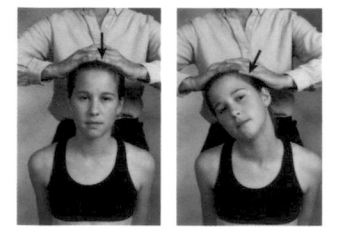

CERVICAL FORAMINAL DISTRACTION TEST

Purpose: Assess cervical mobility, foraminal size, & nerve root impingement

Position: Supine or sitting

Technique: Clinician imparts a controlled distraction force of the C-spine to ↑ the IVF space & decompress the facet jts

Interpretation: + test = ↓ or centralization of symptoms implies an effective means of intervention; pain = spinal ligament tear, annulus fibrosis tear/inflammation, large disk herniation, muscle guarding

Statistics: Sensitivity = 40%–44% & specificity = 90%–100%

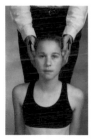

VERTEBRAL ARTERY TEST

Purpose: Test for integrity of internal carotid arteries

Position: Supine

Technique: Place hands under client's occiput to passively extend & SB C-spine then rotate to ~45° & hold x 30 sec; engage client in conversation while monitoring pupils & affect; repeat with rotation to opposite direction

Interpretation: + test = occlusion of vertebral artery inhibits normal blood flow & may result in nausea, dizziness, diplopia, tinnitus, confusion, nystagmus, unilateral pupil changes

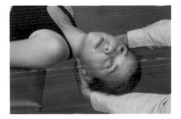

ALAR LIGAMENT TEST

Purpose: Assess alar ligament integrity

Position: Supine

Technique: While palpating spinous process (SP) of C2, slightly SB head

Interpretation: Under normal conditions, (R) rotation & SB tightens (L) alar ligament & flexion tightens both. Thus, the SP should move immediately in the contralateral direction to SB (+) test = a delay in SP movement of C2 may indicate pathology of the alar ligament (most common in client's with RA)

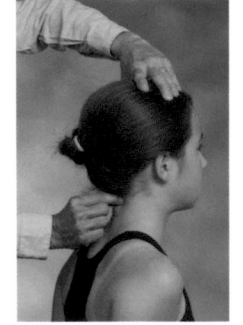

TRANSVERSE LIGAMENT TEST

Purpose: Assess transverse portion of cruciform ligament

Position: Supine with head cradled in the clinician's hands

Technique: Anterior & posterior glides are used to locate the anterior arches of C2. Once identified, the C2 arches are stabilized posteriorly with the clinician's thumbs & the client's occiput is lifted with the cupped hands to translate the head forward. This glides the head & C1 anterior on C2. Hold for 15-30 seconds

Interpretation: + test = Vertigo, nystagmus, paresthesia into face or UE & indicates A-A instability 2° pathology of transverse ligament

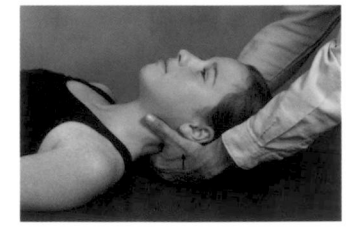

LATERAL & AP RIB COMPRESSION

Purpose. Assess ribs for fx

Position: Supine

Technique: With clinician's hands on the lateral aspect of the rib cage, compress bilaterally; repeat with hands on the front & back of the chest

Interpretation: + test = pain due to rib fracture or costochondral separation

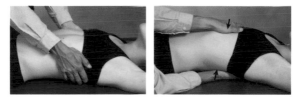

RIB MOTION TEST

Purpose: Assess costal mobility

Position: Supine

Technique: Palpate AP mov't of ribs as client inhales/exhales

Interpretation: During inspiration, ribs 1–6 should ↑ in AP dimension, while ribs 7–10 should ↑ in lateral dimension via bucket handle action & ribs 8–12 should ↑ in lateral dimension via caliper action; ι test – inhibited rib movement with exhalation suggests an elevated rib; inhibited rib movement with inhalation suggests a depressed rib

BEEVOR'S SIGN

Purpose: Assess abdominal musculature

Position: Supine with knees flexed & feet on mat

Technique: Head & shoulders are raised off the mat while movement of the umbilicus is observed

Interpretation: Umbilicus should remain in a straight line. + test depends on direction of movement. Movement distally = weak upper abdominals, movement proximally = weak lower abdominals, movement up & (R) = weak muscles in (L) lower quadrant, movement down & (L) = weak muscles in the (R) upper quadrant

QUADRATUS TEST
Purpose: Assess quadratus lumborum muscle strength
Position: Ipsilateral side-lying on elbow
Technique: Lift ipsilateral hip to align back & lower extremities
Interpretation: + test = inability to lift hip = weakness

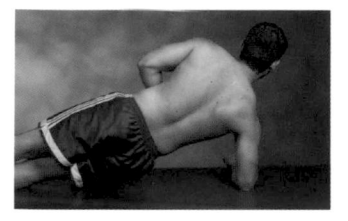

STANDING / SITTING FORWARD FLEXION TEST
Purpose: Assess mobility of ilium or sacrum
Position: Standing or sitting
Technique: Palpate PSIS while client slowly FB with LE straight & hands reaching toward the floor
Interpretation: Segmental movement should begin with L-spine, then sacrum, & then innominate; (+) test = asymmetrical movement with the pathologic side being the one that moves more
Statistics: Sensitivity = 17% & specificity = 79%

GILLET'S MARCH TEST
Purpose: Assess innominate mobility
Position: Standing
Technique: While clinician palpates inferior aspect of (R) PSIS with 1 thumb & medial sacral crest (S2 @ the level of the PSIS) with 1 thumb, client is asked to flex the (R) hip to 90°–120°; repeat other side
Interpretation: Normal = L-spine (L) SB & (R) rotation should be accompanied by (R) innominate rotating posterior & sacrum rotating (L); + test = asymmetrical PSIS movement, pop/click, or reproduction of pain
Statistics: Sensitivity = 8%–43% & specificity = 68%–93%

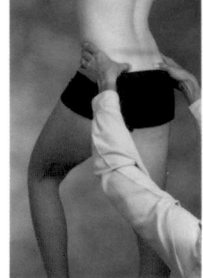

SUPINE TO SIT TEST

Purpose: Assess position of the ilium

Position: Supine with both LEs extended

Technique: Palpate medial malleolus as client performs a long sit-up (Be careful not to rotate the trunk while sitting up)

Interpretation: + test = a short-to-long leg position = posterior ilium rotation; a long-to-short leg position = anterior ilium rotation

Statistics: Sensitivity = 44% & specificity = 64%

LUMBAR QUADRANT TEST

Purpose: Assess nerve roots & IVF

Position: Standing or sitting

Technique: Assist the client in extending spine & SB ipsilaterally with rotation contralaterally & then apply overpressure through the shoulders; repeat to other side

Interpretation: + test = radicular symptoms are due to nerve root compression whereas local pain incriminates the facet joints

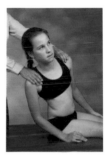

PRONE KNEE BENDING

Purpose: Assess neural mobility

Position: Basic test position = prone with hips extended

Technique: Add each of the following motions to implicate a specific nerves.

Interpretation: + test = reproduction of symptoms

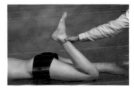

Modification for nerve bias:	Nerve implicated:
Knee flexion	Femoral nerve (L2–4)
Hip adduction with knee flexion	Lateral femoral cutaneous nerve
Hip abduction, ER, knee extension, & ankle dorsiflexion & eversion	Saphenous nerve

SLR TEST

Purpose: Assess neural mobility

Position: Basic SLR test position = hip flexion, adduction, IR with knee extended

Technique: Add each of the following motions to implicate specific nerves

Modification for nerve bias:	Nerve implicated:
Dorsiflexion	Sciatic nerve
Dorsiflexion, eversion, & toe extension	Tibial nerve
Dorsiflexion & inversion	Sural nerve
Plantarflexion & inversion	Common peroneal nerve

Interpretation: + test = reproduction of symptoms

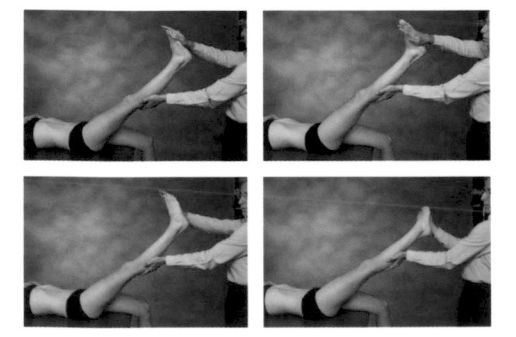

Statistics: Sensitivity = 76%–96% & specificity = 10%–45%

STOOP TEST

Purpose: Differentiate neurogenic vs. vascular intermittent claudication

Position: Standing

Technique: Client walks briskly until symptoms appear & then flexes forward or sits

Interpretation: + test = if symptoms are quickly relieved with FB, claudication is neurogenic; can also perform on a stationary bike

SI POSTERIOR COMPRESSION TEST (Anterior Gapping)

Purpose: Assess for SI pathology

Position: Supine with clinician's hands crossed over client's pelvis on ASISs

Technique: Apply a lateral force to the ASISs through the hands

Interpretation: + test = reproduction of SI joint pain

Statistics: Sensitivity = 7%–69% & specificity = 69%–100%

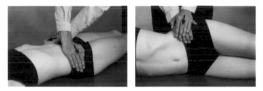

SI POSTERIOR GAPPING TEST (Compression of iliac crests)

Purpose: Assess for SI pathology

Position: Side-lying

Technique: Apply a downward force through the anterior aspect of the ASIS to create posterior gapping of the SI

Interpretation: + test = reproduction of SI joint pain

Statistics: Sensitivity = 4%–60% & specificity = 81%–100%

HOOVER TEST

Purpose: Assess malingering

Position: Supine

Technique: Hold client's heels of (B) LEs in clinician's hands, ask client to lift 1 leg out of a hand

Interpretation: + test = client does not lift the leg & there is no downward force exerted by the contralateral limb

SI Cluster Tests	Sensitivity	Specificity
• Standing flexion, PSIS palpation, supine to long-sit, & prone knee flexion	82	88
• Distraction, thigh thrust, compression, & sacral thrust	91	78
• Thigh thrust, distraction, sacral thrust, & compression	88	78

Waddell Nonorganic Signs

Sign	Description
Tenderness—superficial or nonanatomic	Tenderness is not related to a particular structure. It may be superficial (tender to a light pinch over a wide area) or deep tenderness felt over a wide area (may extend over many segmental levels).
Simulation tests—axial loading in rotation	These tests give the client the impression that diagnostic tests are being performed. Slight pressure (axial loading) applied to the top of the head or passive rotation of the shoulders & pelvis in the same direction produces c/o LBP
Distraction tests – SLR	A (+) clinical test (SLR) is confirmed by testing the structures in another position. By appearing to test the plantar reflex in sitting, the examiner may actually lift the leg higher than that of the supine SLR.
Regional disturbances—weakness or sensory	When the dysfunction spans a widespread region of the body (sensory or motor) that cannot be explained via anatomical relationships. This may be demonstrated by the client "giving way" or cogwheel resistance during strength testing of many major muscle groups or reporting diminish sensation in a nondermatomal pattern (stocking effect)
Overreaction	Disproportionate responses via verbalization, facial expressions, muscle tremors, sweating, collapsing, rubbing affected area, or emotional reactions.

Note: Any positive test in 3 or more categories results in an overall Waddell Score.

Differential Diagnosis

Pathology/Mechanism	Signs/Symptoms
Torticollis—7 forms of congenital torticollis & other causes include hemivertebra, cervical pharyngitis (major cause in 5–10 yo), JRA, trauma	■ Symptoms appear @ 6–8 weeks of age ■ ↓ Contralateral rotation & ipsilateral SB (unilateral) ■ Firm, nontender swelling about the size of an adult thumb nail ■ (−) x-ray ■ Complications include visual issues &/or reflux
Cervical Sprain—trauma or prolonged static positioning	■ Localized pain; TTP; protective muscle guarding ■ MTrP in cervical, shoulder, & scapular regions ■ ↓ Cervical ROM & stiffness with activity ■ Headache & postural changes—forward head, kyphosis ■ Screen for alar & transverse ligament px ■ Clear vertebral arteries ■ Normal DTRs & (−) x-ray
Cervical Strain—single traumatic event or cumulative trauma; most often occurs in 20–40 yo who have faulty posture, overweight, deconditioning	■ Pain with contraction & with stretching ■ Pain with prolonged sitting, walking, standing ■ TTP & protective muscle guarding ■ Pain appears several hours after injury; headache ■ ↓ Contralateral SB & rotation (AROM <PROM) ■ Clear vertebral arteries ■ Normal DTRs ■ (−) special tests & (−) x-rays

Continued

Pathology/Mechanism	Signs/Symptoms
Cervical Stenosis—most common 30–60 yo; ♂ > ♀; can be congenital or developmental, onset is gradual	■ Unilateral or bilateral symptoms usually span several dermatomes ■ ↑ Pain with cervical BB & ↓ with cervical FB ■ Pain relieved with rest ■ Loss of hand dexterity, LOB & unsteady gait ■ (+) Quadrant test ■ LMN signs at the level of the stenosis & UMN signs below the level of stenosis ■ X-rays reveal spondylitic bars & osteophytes & ossification of PLL & Ligamentum Flavum
Cervical Spondylosis—↑ onset with aging but may be accelerated by cumulative trauma, poor body mechanics, postural changes, or previous disk injury; most common @ C5–7	■ ↑ Pain with activity & stiffness @ rest ■ Limited A & PROM; crepitus ■ (+) Compression/distraction test ■ ↓ Disk height on x-ray; need to r/o osteophytes
Cervical Disk Pathology (most common level is C5–6)—usually the result of repetitive stresses on the neck as a result of poor posture or muscle imbalances; most common in 30–50 yo	■ (+) NTPT—median nerve with contralateral cervical SB, cervical rotation <60° & cervical FB <50° ■ (+) Tests: compression, distraction, shoulder depression & Spurling's maneuver ■ Sensory changes in the respective dermatome ■ X-rays are of little value ■ CT & MRI used to differentiate nucleus pulposus from annulus fibrosis
Cervical Facet Syndrome—occurs as a result of isolated or cumulative trauma, DDD, aging, or postural imbalances	■ Pain with hyperextension & rotation of c-spine ■ Muscle guarding & stiffness ■ Poor movement patterns but no weakness ■ Paresthesia but no changes in DTRs ■ Possible (+) NTPT; (+) Quadrant test ■ (–) X-ray

Continued

Pathology/Mechanism	Signs/Symptoms
Brachial Plexus Lesion (Plexopathy, Burner, Stinger)—occurs from stretching or compression of C-spine or forceful depression of shoulder	■ Sharp & burning pain in UE ■ Numbness/pins & needles present in UE ■ Transient muscle weakness & ↓ DTR ■ Provocation test = ipsilateral cervical SB with compression OR contralateral SB (stretch) ■ (+) NTPT ■ Confirmed with myelogram
Rib Fracture—mechanism is a direct blow; cough in a frail person	■ (+) Tests: AP & lateral rib compression ■ TTP & pain with deep inspiration ■ (+) X-ray is difficult to assess immediately after injury
Costochondritis—may be due to trauma, infection, arthritis, or surgery	■ Localized pain in anterior chest wall ■ TTP; pain ↑ with cough that may radiate into UE
Compression Fracture—most common in T11–L2, may be related to trauma or osteoporosis	■ Acute pain with adjacent muscle guarding ■ Limited BB & rotation ■ (+) X-ray
Spondylosis / Arthrosis—degenerative changes that usually effects C5–6, C6–7, L4–5 of clients >60 yo	■ Onset is slow; pain is unilateral & ↑ with prolonged postures ■ Pain ↑ with BB & ↓ with FB but usually does not radiate ■ Confirmed with x-ray; osteophytes, ↓ joint space, & narrow IVF may be present
Spondylolysis—traumatic fractures of pars or stress fractures due to repeated or sustained extension, seen in young athletes 2° repetitive trauma (ski jumping, gymnastics); may have a structural predisposition	■ Pain primarily with extension ■ Intermittent neurologic signs & symptoms ■ Oblique x-ray reveals fracture of pars interarticularis without slippage (Scottie dog with a collar)

Continued

Continued

Pathology/Mechanism	Signs/Symptoms
Spondylolisthesis—vertebral subluxation or slippage 2° a long history of LB trauma Retrolisthesis = not common but presents with flexion symptoms	■ L5 nerve entrapment → sciatica ■ Morning stiffness; difficulty getting OOB ■ ↑ Pain with trunk extension ■ Poor neuromuscular control— ■ "Hitching sign" = 2-step process of moving from FB & BB via 1st extending lumbar spine into lordosis & then extending hip ■ Palpable step deformity in WB, gone in NWB ■ (+) Tests: PIVM & compression test ■ A/P & lateral x-ray confirms dx
Lumbar Disk Pathology—usually the result of repetitive stresses on the LB using improper body mechanics or excessive force posterior/lateral > lateral; most common in 30–50 yo **Note:** See "Lumbar Disk Posturing & Pain" on page 173.	*Posterior-lateral HNP:* ■ 1st sign is LBP that slowly diminishes to leg pain ■ LB flexion 2° ↑ disk pressure ■ (+) Thecal signs (pain with sneezing & coughing) ■ (+) SLR; ↑ lumbar lordosis ■ Lateral shift in standing that ↑ in supine *Lateral HNP:* ■ No LBP, LE symptoms consistent with level of injury ■ ↓ Pain with standing & walking; ↑ with sitting ■ (−) SLR ■ Standard x-rays are of little value because they may only detect pre-existing degenerative changes; MRI, CT scan, myelogram & discogram are used for diagnosis
Lumbar Sprain—usually results from a combination of forward bending with rotation in SB; common in people <30 yo	■ Unilateral LBP ■ Pain with SB away & rotation toward affected side ■ Referred pain to gluteals & thigh regions

Pathology/Mechanism	Signs/Symptoms
Lumbar Facet Syndrome—occurs as a result of isolated or cumulative trauma, DDD, aging, or postural imbalances	■ Pain referred to gluteals or thigh ■ Muscle guarding ■ Pain primarily with compression; morning stiffness ■ Pain ↓ with FB ■ Pain ↑ with BB & ipsilateral SB; difficulty standing straight ■ X-ray may show osteophytes (spondylosis)
Lumbar Stenosis—progressive, irreversible, & insidious onset of narrowing of the spinal canal; history of LBP × several years; occurs mostly in people over 50 yo; ♂ > ♀	■ Dull ache across LS region when standing & walking ■ ↓ Pain when leaning forward, walking uphill, with pillow under knees, knees to chest, or sitting in flexion ■ Usually (B) pain into buttocks & proximal thigh ■ Nocturnal pain & cramping ■ Paresthesia that ↑ with BB & WB ■ (–) Tests: SLR & femoral nerve test ■ Postural changes: ↓ Lumbar lordosis & LE flexion ■ No change in B&B or pulses ■ LMN signs at level of lesion, UMN signs below level of lesion (ataxia, reflex hyperactivity (3+), (+) stoop test, & proprioceptive deficits) ■ X-ray may show osteophytes or ossification of PLL & ligamentum flavum; CT scan may show bony encroachment of spinal canal; MRI confirms clinical findings; myelogram will show amount of constriction of thecal sac

Continued

Pathology/Mechanism	Signs/Symptoms
Trochanteric Bursitis—may result from contralateral gluteus medius weakness or a change/↑ in activity level; direct trauma	■ Pain into buttock & lateral thigh ■ Pain worse at night & with activity ■ TTP over greater trochanter ■ Possible "clicking" with AROM & pain with resisted hip abduction ■ Check for leg length discrepancy ■ (−) X-ray
Piriformis Syndrome—most commonly due to repeated compressive forces or may result from a change/↑ in activity level; ♀ > ♂	■ Piriformis TTP ■ Ipsilateral LB, buttock, & referred LE pain ■ Pain & weakness with resisted abduction/ER of thigh ■ Pain with stretch into hip flexion, adduction & IR ■ (−) X-ray; need to r/o sprain/strain or HNP
Ischiogluteal Bursitis—may result from a change/↑ in activity level	■ Pain into buttock & posterior thigh that is worse in sitting ■ TTP over ischial tuberosity ■ (+) Tests: SLR & Patrick test ■ (−) X-ray

Ankylosing Spondylitis (Marie Stüumpell's disease)—involves anterior longitudinal ligament & ossification of disk & thoracic zygapophyseal joints; most common in 15–40 yo; ♂ > ♀	■ Postural changes:
	  ■ Cervical hyperextension
	  ■ Thoracic kyphosis
	  ■ ↓ Lumbar lordosis
	  ■ Hip & knee flexion contractures
	■ Night pain & ↓ rib expansion
	■ ↑ SED rate
	■ 5 screening questions:
	  ■ Morning stiffness > 30 minutes
	  ■ Improvement with exercise
	  ■ Onset of back pain before 40 yo
	  ■ Slow onset
	  ■ Symptoms >3 months
	4+ positive questions is highly correlated with AS

Continued

Pathology/Mechanism	Signs/Symptoms
Osteoporosis—results from insufficient formation or excessive resorption of bone; occurs with ↑ age, low body fat, low Ca++ intake, high caffeine intake, bed rest, alcoholism, steroid use	■ Dowager's hump (dorsal kyphosis) ■ Loss of height (2–4 cm/fracture) ■ Acute regional back pain (low thoracic/high lumbar) ■ Pain radiating anterior along costal margins ■ Fragile skin ■ X-ray does not show bone loss but will reveal fx ■ Bone scan needed for confirmation

Vascular vs. Neurological Claudication

Vascular Signs & Symptoms		Neurogenical Signs & Symptoms
Primarily affects people >40 yo	**Population**	
Bilateral—hip, thigh, & buttock to calf	**Pain location**	Unilateral or bilateral—LB & buttocks
Cramping, aching, squeezing	**Pain description**	Numbness, tingling, burning, weakness
Pain is present regardless of spinal position	**Positional response**	Pain ↓ with spinal flexion & ↑ with spinal extension
Pain brought on by physical exertion (walking, particularly uphill) & relieved within minutes of rest	**Response to activity**	Pain ↑ with walking & ↓ with recumbency
↓ LE pulses; color & skin changes	**Pulses & skin**	Normal pulses & skin
No burning or sensation changes	**Sensation**	Burning & numbness in LE

Lumbar Disk Posturing & Pain

Posturing	PAIN	
	Herniation medial to nerve root	Herniation lateral to nerve root
Ipsilateral list (medial pain behavior)	↑ Pain	↓ Pain
Contralateral list (lateral pain behavior)	↓ Pain	↑ Pain

Prognosis of a Lumbar Disk Herniation

Factors that can influence a (+) outcome:		Factors that can influence a (−) outcome
■ (−) Crossed SLR test ■ No leg pain with spinal extension ■ Large extrusion or sequestration ■ (+) Response to corticosteroids ■ Progressive recovery of neurological deficits in first 12 weeks	Clinical	■ (+) Crossed SLR test ■ Leg pain with spinal extension ■ Contained herniation ■ (−) Response to corticosteroids ■ Presence of spinal stenosis ■ Progressive neurological deficit ■ Cauda equina syndrome
■ Limited psychosocial issues ■ Self-employed ■ Motivated ■ >12 years of education ■ Good fitness level ■ No Waddell's signs	Psychosocial	■ Overbearing psychosocial issues ■ Worker's compensation ■ Unmotivated ■ <12 years of education ■ Illiterate ■ >3 Waddell's signs

Differential Diagnosis of Sacroiliac Dysfunctions

Diagnosis	Sacral Base	ILA	Lumbar Spine	Seated Flexion Test	Sit-Slump Test	Sacral Spring Test
(R)Sacral flexion	Deep (R)	Shallow (R) Caudal (R)	Convex (R)	(+) (R)	Deep (R) base with slump	← (R)ILA spring on MTA
(L)Sacral flexion	Deep (L)	Shallow (L) Caudal (L)	Convex (L)	(+) (L)	Deep (L) base with slump	← (L)ILA spring on MTA
Bilateral sacral flexion	Deep (B)	Deep (B)	↓ Lordosis			
(R)Sacral extension	Shallow (R)	Deep (R) Cranial (R)	Convex (L)	(+) (R)	Shallow (R) base with ext	← (R)sacral base on MTA
(L)Sacral extension	Shallow (L)	Deep (L) Cranial (L)	Convex (R)	(+) (L)	Shallow (L) base with ext	← left sacral base on MTA
Bilateral sacra extension	Shallow (B)	Deep (B)	↑ Lordosis			
(L)/(L)FW sacral torsion	Deep (R)	Shallow (R) Caudal (R)	Convex (L)	(+) (R)	Shallow (R) base with ext	← (L)ILA spring on LOA
(R)/(R)FW sacral torsion	Deep (L)	Shallow (L) Caudal (L)	Convex (R)	(+) (L)	Deep (L) base with slump	← (R)ILA spring on ROA
(L)/(R)BW sacral torsion	Deep (L)	Deep (R) Caudal (R)	Convex (L)	(+) (R)	Shallow (L) base with ext	← (L)sacral base on ROA
(R)/(L)BW sacral torsion	Shallow (R)	Deep (L) Caudal (L)	Convex (L)	(+) (R)	Shallow (R) base w/h ext	← (R)sacral base on LOA

ILA = inferior lateral angle
LOA = left oblique axis

ROA = right oblique axis
MTA = middle transverse axis

Differential Diagnosis of Iliosacral Dysfunctions

Diagnosis	Etiology	SFT	ASIS	PSIS	Sacral sulcus	Soft tissue TTP	Leg length
(R) Anterior Innominate	Weak glut med/max or abdominals, golf	(+) (R)	(R) Low	(R) high	(R) Shallow	Left TFL	(R) Shortens with long sitting
(R) Posterior Innominate	Prolonged (R) LE WB, fall on (R) ischium, weak (R) glut med, tight hamstrings, short (R) leg	(+) (R)	(R) Up & forward	(R) Down & back	(L) Deep	(R) Piriformis & TFL	(R) Leg lengthens with long sitting
(R) Inflare	Muscle Imbalances, weak (R) glut med	(+) (R)	(R) Medial	(R) Lateral	(R) Wider	(R) Piriformis	
(R) Outflare	Muscle imbalances	(+) (R)	(R) Lateral	(R) Medial	(R) Narrow		
(R) Upslip innominate			(R) High	(R) High			

Continued

Differential Diagnosis of Iliosacral Dysfunctions—cont'd

Diagnosis	Etiology	SFT	ASIS	PSIS	Sacral sulcus	Soft tissue TTP	Leg length
Ⓕ Downslip innominate			Ⓡ Low	Ⓡ Low			
Ⓡ Superior pubic shear	Fall on ischium or landing on 1 leg	(+) Ⓡ	Poss. Ⓡ high	Poss. Ⓡ high	Ⓡ shallow	Tight ITB, adductors & Ⓡ quadratus TTP	Supine to sit = short to long
Ⓡ Inferior pubic shear	Short leg, weak glut medius &/or tight ITB	(+) Ⓡ	Poss. Ⓡ low	Poss. Ⓡ low		SIJ TTP	

SFT = Standing Flexion Test
ASIS = Anterior Superior Iliac Spine
PSIS = Posterior Superior Iliac Spine
TTP = Tender To Palpation

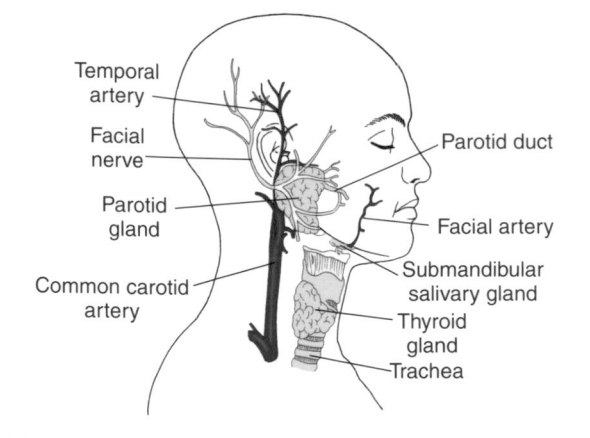

Temporal artery

Facial nerve

Parotid gland

Common carotid artery

Parotid duct

Facial artery

Submandibular salivary gland

Thyroid gland

Trachea

Ligaments of the jaw

Sphenomandibular ligament

Zygomatic arch

Joint capsule

Lateral (temporomandibular) ligament

Styloid process

Stylomandibular ligament

176

Referral Patterns

Muscle Pain Referral Patterns

Masseter · Sternocleidomastoid

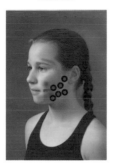 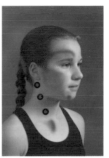

Scalene muscle

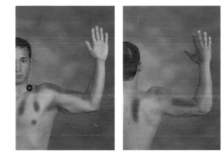

Digastric

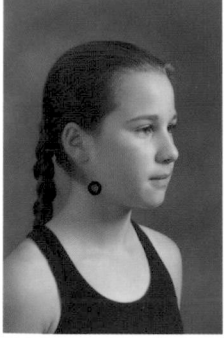
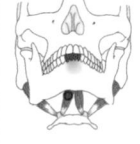

Temporalis

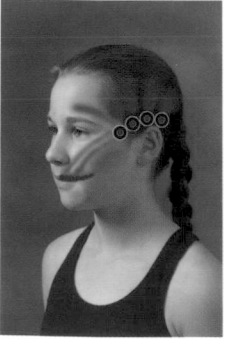

Medial & lateral pterygoid

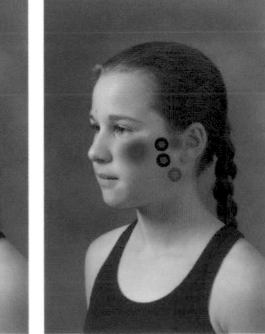

Palpation Pearls

- **SCM**—in supine, find mastoid process & move toward the clavicular notch, have client raise head & slightly rotate to opposite side
- **Scalenes**—stringy muscle above the clavicle between the SCM & traps; to confirm identification, palpate in the general area & have client inhale deeply & scalenes should be in the middle of the triangle
- **Masseter**—palpate the side of the mandible between the zygomatic arch & the angle of the mandible, have client clench the jaw
- **Suprahyoids**—palpate under the tip of the chin & resist mandibular depression or have the client swallow to confirm identification
- **Anterior digastric**—palpate extraorally inferior to body of the mandible
- **Posterior digastric**—palpate extraorally posterior to the angle of the mandible
- **Medial pterygoid**—palpate intraorally along medial rim of the mandible
- **Lateral pterygoid**—palpate intraorally along superior, posterior aspect behind 3rd maxillary molar

ROM

- Mandibular depression (opening)—35–50 mm (2–3 knuckles) is functional

  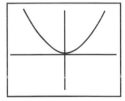

  - C-deviation = hypomobility toward side of deviation (lateral pterygoid tension or disk pathology)
  - S-deviation = muscle imbalance or displacement of condyle around disk
- Mandibular elevation (closing)—palpate quality of movement to resting position
- Mandibular protrusion = 6–9 mm; must take into account the starting position if there is an overbite or underbite present
- Mandibular retrusion = 3–4 mm
- Mandibular lateral excursion = 10–15 mm

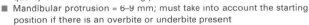

Osteokinematics of the TMJ

Motion	Normal End-feel(s)	Abnormal End-feel(s)
Opening/ Closing	Open = tissue stretch/elastic Closed = bone-to-bone	Hard = osseous abnormality
Protrusion/ retrusion	Tissue stretch/elastic	Springy = disk displacement
Lateral excursion	Tissue stretch/elastic	Capsular = shortening of periarticular tissues

Arthrokinematics of TMJ

Opening & closing	**Concave surface:** Mandibular fossa **Convex surface:** Mandibular condyle & disk	*To facilitate opening:* Condyles rotate anterior for the first 25°, then anterior & inferior gliding of condyle & disk completes the last 15° of movement	*To facilitate closing:* Condyles & disk roll posterior & glide medially & superior
Protrusion & retrusion	**Concave surface:** Mandibular fossa **Convex surface:** Mandibular condyle & disk	*To facilitate protrusion:* Disk & condyle move down & FW	*To facilitate retrusion:* Disk & condyle move up & BW
Lateral excursion	**Concave surface:** Mandibular fossa **Convex surface:** Mandibular condyle & disk	*To facilitate lateral excursion:* (R) excursion = (L) condyle & disk glide anterior; while (R) condyle spins around vertical axis (L) excursion = (R) condyle & disk glide anterior; while (L) condyle spins around vertical axis	

Special Tests

- **CLEAR CRANIAL NERVES** – see "Alerts/Alarms" tab page 13.
- **AUSCULTATION**—used to identify poor joint kinematics or joint/disk damage; place stethoscope over TMJ, just anterior to tragus of ear, and clinician listens for presence of joint sounds; very sensitive to finding a problem but not specific in the identification of the structure.

Interpretation:
  - Opening click = click as condyle moves over posterior aspect of disk in an effort to restore normal relationship; disk is anterior to condyle; the later the click, the more anterior the disk
  - Reciprocal click = in opening, the disk reduces as the condyle moves under the disk & in closing, a second click is heard as the condyle slips posteriorly & the disk becomes displaced anteriorly

LATERAL POLE
Purpose: Assess soft tissues of TMJ
Position: Face client with clinician's index fingers palpating lateral pole of TMJ
Technique: Open & close mouth several times
Interpretation: + test = $\uparrow$ or reproduction of symptoms incriminating LCL or TMJ ligament

EXTERNAL AUDITORY MEATUS
Purpose: Assess posterior disk
Position: Face client, clinician inserts little fingers into client's ears
Technique: While applying forward pressure with fingers, client opens & closes mouth repeatedly
Interpretation: + test – $\uparrow$ or reproduction of symptoms
Statistics: Sensitivity = 43% & specificity = 75%

DYNAMIC LOADING
Purpose: To mimic TMJ loading to differentiate between TMJ & muscle pain
Position: Sitting with roll of gauze between molars on 1-side
Technique: Client bites down on gauze roll
Interpretation: Compression occurs on contralateral side & distraction on ipsilateral side of gauze; + test – $\uparrow$ or reproduction of symptoms @ TMJ

Pathology/Mechanism	Signs/Symptoms
Inflammation—may be the result of acute or repetitive trauma, prolonged immobilization or surgery	■ Capsular tightness with ↓ opening ■ Pain with or without movement ■ Need to r/o disk displacement
***Disk Displacement**—may be related to poor posture, trauma, excessive opening, muscle imbalance (anterior displacement is most common)	■ Muscle guarding ■ Localized TTP ■ Headache ■ Confirmed with MRI
TMJ Arthritis—gradual onset, poor kinematics or repeated trauma of the TMJ that leads to joint erosion	■ Pain, stiffness, crepitus, clicking, grinding ■ ↓ ROM (deviation toward involved side) ■ Headache ■ Hearing loss & dizziness ■ Confirmed with x-ray or MRI; need to r/o disk problem

*Disk can result in clicking or locking. Locked open = disk is anterior and with opening there is a click with the disk being displaced posterior, then the joint is locked in the open position; locked closed = disk is anterior to the condyle so anterior translation is limited & opening is reduced.

Anatomy of the Hip

Muscles of the hip

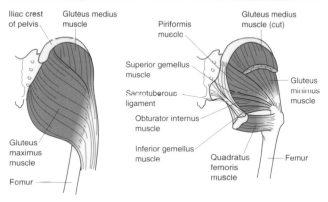

Palpation Pearls

Femoral triangle

- Superior border = inguinal ligament
- Lateral to medial = sartorius, femoral nerve, femoral artery, femoral vein, great saphenous vein, pectineus muscle, & adductor longus muscle
- Piriformis – find mid-point between PSIS & coccyx, piriformis runs from this point lateral to greater trochanter

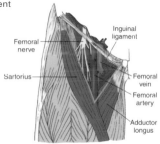

Medical Red Flags

- Pain @ McBurney's point = ⅓–½ the distance from (R) ASIS to umbilicus; tenderness = appendicitis
- Blumberg's sign = rebound tenderness for visceral pathology—in supine select a site away from the painful area, place your hand perpendicular to the abdomen & push down deep & slow; lift up quickly; (–) = no pain; (+) = pain on release
- Psoas test for pelvic pathology = supine, SLR to 30° & resist hip flexion; (+) test for pelvic inflammation or infection in lower quadrant abdominal pain; hip or back pain is a (–) test
- Constitutional symptoms
- Enlarged inguinal lymph nodes
- Hip pain in men 18–24 years old of unknown etiology should be screened for testicular CA
- Systemic causes of hip pain
    - Bone tumors
    - Crohn's disease
    - Inflammatory bowel or pelvic inflammatory disease
    - Ankylosing spondylitis
    - Sickle cell anemia
    - Hemophilia
    - Urogenital problems
- Neuromusculoskeletal causes of hip pain
    - LB &/or SI
    - OA or stress fx
    - Hernia
    - Muscle weakness
    - Sprain/strain
    - Labral tear
- Screen for a sports hernia
    - Palpation of marble-sized lump along the path of the inguinal ligament
    - Pain with exertion, cough, menstruation
    - Radiating pain into groin, ipsilateral thigh, flank, or lower abdomen
    - Pain with cutting, turning, striding out

Toolbox Tests

Western Ontario & McMaster Universities Osteoarthritis Index (WOMAC)

Instructions: Please rate the activities in each category according to the following scale of difficulty:
0 = none; 1 = slight; 2 = moderate; 3 = very; 4 = extremely

Pain	· Walking	
	· Stair climbing	
	· Nocturnal	
	· Rest	
	· Weight bearing	
Stiffness	· Morning stiffness	
	· Stiffness occurring later in the day	
Physical Function	· Descending stairs	
	· Ascending stairs	
	· Rising from sitting	
	· Standing	
	· Bending to floor	
	· Walking on flat surface	
	· Getting in/out of car	
	· Going shopping	
	· Putting on socks	
	· Lying in bed	
	· Taking off socks	
	· Rising from bed	
	· Getting in/out of bath	
	· Sitting	
	· Getting on/off toilet	
	· Heavy domestic duties	
	· Light domestic duties	
Total Score		

Scoring: Summate the scores of each item for the total score. The higher the score, the more severe the disability.

Source: From Bellamy, et al. Journal of Rheumatology, 15:1833–1840, 1988.

HARRIS Hip Score

Select the descriptor for each section that best describes your current condition

Pain—44 possible points

None or ignores it	44
Slight, occasional, no compromise in activities	40
Mild pain, no effect on average activities, moderate pain with unusual activities, may take aspirin	30
Moderate pain, tolerable but makes concessions, some limitation of ordinary activity, occasional pain medicine stronger than aspirin	20
Marked pain, serious limitation of activity	10
Totally disabled, crippled, pain in bed, bedridden	0

Function/Gait—33 possible points

Distance Walked	Unlimited	11
	4–6 blocks	8
	2–3 blocks	5
	Indoors only	2
	Unable to walk	0
Limp	None	11
	Slight	8
	Moderate	5
	Severe	0
Support	None	11
	Cane for long walks	7
	Cane most of the time	5
	One crutch	3
	Two canes	2
	Two crutches	0
	Not able to walk	0

Continued

HARRIS Hip Score—*cont'd*

Select the descriptor for each section that best describes your current condition

Function/Activities—14 possible points		
Stairs	Normally without rail	4
	Normally with rail	2
	In any manner	1
	Unable to do stairs	0
Shoes & Socks	With ease	4
	With difficulty	2
	Unable	0
Sitting	Comfortable in ordinary chair 1 hr	5
	On a high chair for ½ hr	3
	Unable to sit comfortably	0
Enter Public Transportation		1

Deformity—4 points for each of the following present	
<30° flexion contracture	
<10° adduction contracture	
<10° abduction contracture	
<3.2 cm leg-length discrepancy	

ROM		
Flexion	0–45° (1.0 point per degree)	
	+ 0.6 points/degree from 45°–90°	
	+ 0.3 points/degree from 90°–110°	
Abduction	0–15° (0.8 points per degree)	
	+ 0.3 points/degree from 15°–20°	
ER (in ext)	0–15° (0.4 points per degree)	
Adduction	0–15° (0.2 points per degree)	
Total Score		

Scoring: The higher the total score, the lower the level of disability.

Source: From Harris, WH. Journal of Bone and Joint Surgery, 51-A(4):737–755, 1969.

Referral Patterns

Muscle Pain Referral Patterns

Iliopsoas

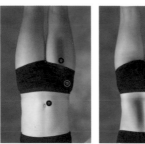

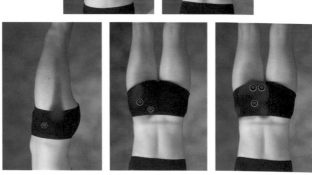

Tensor fascia latae

Piriformis

Gluteus maximus

Osteokinematics of the Hip

Normal ROM	OPP	CPP	Normal End-feel(s)	Abnormal End-feel(s)
Flexion = 100°–120° Ext = 15° Abduction = 40°–45° IR = 30°–40° ER = 40°–50°	30° flexion 30° abd & slight FR	max ext, IR, abd	Flexion & Add = elastic or tissue approx SLR = elastic Ext & Abd = elastic/firm IR & ER = elastic/firm	Capsular = IR > Ext > Abd

Arthrokinematics for Hip Mobilization

Concave surface: acetabulum	*To facilitate hip flexion:* Femur spins posterior	*To facilitate hip extension:* Femur spins anterior
	To facilitate hip abduction: Femur spins lateral & glides medial	*To facilitate hip adduction:* Femur spins medial & glides lateral
Convex surface: femoral head	*To facilitate hip IR:* Femur rolls medial & glides lateral on pelvis	*To facilitate hip ER:* Femur rolls lateral & glides medial on pelvis

Special Tests

THOMAS TEST

Purpose: Assess for tight hip flexors
Position: Supine with lumbar spine stabilized & involved LE extended
Technique: Flex contralateral hip to the abdomen
Interpretation: + test = flexion of the involved hip or lumbar spine indicates tight hip flexors

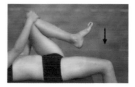

ELY'S TEST

Purpose: Assess for tight rectus femoris
Position: Side-lying or prone, hip in extension
Technique: Flex knee
Interpretation: + test = limited knee flexion with hip extension or inability to maintain hip extension when knee is flexed

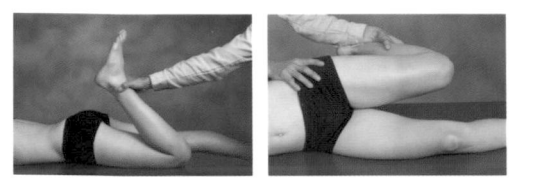

OBER'S TEST

Purpose: Assess for tight ITB
Position: Side-lying with involved hip up
Technique: Extend the involved hip & allow LE to drop into adduction
Interpretation: + test = LE fails to adduct

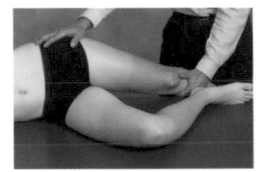

IMPINGEMENT TEST

Purpose: Assess for labral tears & femoroacetabular impingement
Position: Supine
Technique: Simultaneously flex, adduct & ER hip to end range
Interpretation: + test = reproduction of pain
Statistics: Kappa = 0.58

SCOUR TEST

Purpose: Assess for labral tear
Position: Supine, flex hip to 90°
Technique: IR/ER hip with abd/adduction while applying a compressive force down the femur

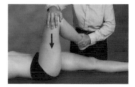

Interpretation: + test = clicking, grinding or pain due to arthritis, acetabular labrum tear, avascular necrosis, or osteochondral defect
Statistics: Sensitivity = 75%–79% & specificity = 43%–50%

ANTERIOR LABRAL TEST

Purpose: Assess for labral tear
Position: Supine in PNF D2 flexion (hip in full flex, ER & abd)
Technique: Resist movement into ext IR & add (D2 extension)
Interpretation: + test = reproduction of pain or click

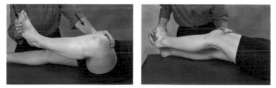

POSTERIOR LABRAL TEST

Purpose: Assess for labral tear
Position: Supine in flexion with adduction, & IR (similar to PNF D1 pattern but with IR)
Technique: Resist movement into ext, abduction, & ER (similar to D1 extension but with ER)
Interpretation: + test = reproduction of pain or click

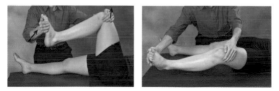

LOG ROLL TEST

Purpose: Assess for iliofemoral ligament laxity

Position: Supine with LEs extended

Technique: Roll the LE into maximal ER by applying a medial to lateral force through the thigh

Interpretation: + test = excessive ER as compared to the contralateral LE

Statistics: Kappa = 0.61

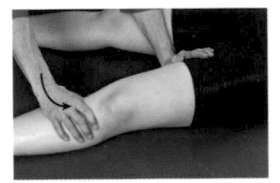

FABER TEST (PATRICK'S)

Purpose: Assess hip/SI & labral pathology

Position: Supine -passively flex, abduct & ER the hip (figure-4 position) so that the lateral malleolus of the involved LE is on the knee of the uninvolved LE

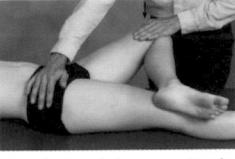

Technique: Apply overpressure to flexed knee

Interpretation: + test = hip pain 2° to OA, osteophytes, intracapsular fx, or LBP 2° SI px; tightness without pain is a (–) test; pain experienced assuming this position may indicate a problem with the sartorius muscle Labral pathology may be suspected if lateral aspect of the knee is >4cm from the surface & asymmetrical

Statistics: Kappa = 0.63; sensitivity = 41%–77%; specificity = 88%–100%

TRENDELENBURG'S TEST

Purpose: Assess for weakness of gluteus medius

Position: Standing on involved LE

Technique: Flex the contralateral LE; iliac crest on WB side should be lower than the NWB side

Interpretation: + test = dropping of the NWB limb is 2° to abductor weakness (common in epiphyseal problem, Legg-Calve-Perthes, MD)

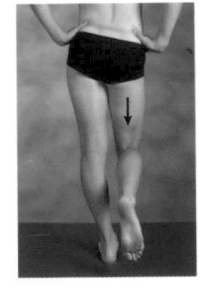

PIRIFORMIS TEST

Purpose: Assess for tight piriformis
Position: Supine or contralateral side-lying
Technique: Flex hip to 70°–80° with knee flexed & maximally adduct LE (apply a downward force to the knee)
Interpretation: + test = pain in buttock & sciatica; IR stresses superior fibers; ER stresses inferior fibers

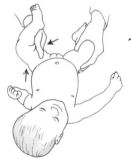

ORTOLANI'S TEST

Purpose: Assess for congenital hip dislocation
Position: Supine fix hips & knees @ 90° of flexion; clinician's thumbs are on the infant's medial thigh & fingers on the lateral thigh
Technique: Firmly traction the thigh while gently abducting the leg so that femoral head is translated anterior into the acetabulum
Interpretation: + test = reduction of the hip; an audible "clunk" may be heard

BARLOW'S TEST

(Opposite of the Ortolani Test)
Purpose: Assess for hip dysplasia
Position: Supine 90/90; clinician's thumbs are on the infant's medial thigh & fingers on the lateral thigh
Technique: Apply a posterior force thru the femur as the thigh is gently adducted
Interpretation: + test = the examiner's finger that is on the greater trochanter will detect a palpable dislocation

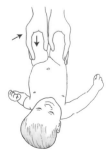

Pathology/Mechanism	Signs/Symptoms
ITB Friction Syndrome—repetitive stress & excessive friction 2° tight ITB, pronation with IR of tibia, genu varum, cycling with cleat in IR Proximal problem = hip syndrome Distal problem = runner's knee	■ Pain with downhill running; sense of knee instability ■ (+) Tests: Ober's, Noble's, & Renne's ■ Pain @ 30° of knee flexion in WB results in ambulating stiff legged to avoid flexion ■ TTP over lateral femoral epicondyle ■ Visible & palpable snapping ■ (−) X-ray; MRI & US may confirm diagnosis ■ Need to r/o trochanteric bursitis & osteochondritis
Greater Trochanteric Bursitis—biomechanical or overuse problem; repetitive inside kicks in soccer result in forceful adduction and compression of bursa; contusions	■ Deep, aching, diffuse pain from greater trochanter to distal lateral thigh & groin ■ TTP on ITB & pain when rolling on hip when sleeping ■ ROM = WNL except abduction may be limited by pain ■ No snapping but palpable crepitus may be present ■ (+) Tests: Ober's & Patrick's/FABER ■ (−) X-ray (needed to r/o femoral neck stress fx) ■ MRI & US may confirm diagnosis
Apophysitis—pelvic fx 2° strenuous muscle contraction in skeletally immature child	■ TTP & weakness with resisted muscle contraction @ ASIS, AIIS, PSIS, PIIS—depending on muscle involved ■ (+) X-ray for avulsion

Continued

Pathology/Mechanism	Signs/Symptoms
Piriformis Syndrome—may result from muscle contracture, trauma, prolonged sitting	■ Dull ache in buttocks ■ Pain ↑ with sitting & walking & ↓ in supine ■ Pain with resisted hip ext & passive IR with adduction ■ (−) X-ray needed to r/o stress fx; MRI needed to r/o spine pathology (LS root lesion, spinal stenosis, SI problem)
Iliopsoas Bursitis/Tendonitis—irritation & inflammation 2° overuse or unaccustomed activity	■ Pain in medial groin/thigh with hip flexion & extension ■ Audible snapping when moving from hip flex to ext ■ Screen for McBurney's point & rebound tenderness ■ (−) X-ray; need to r/o avulsion fx ■ Confirmed by MRI or US
Hip Pointer—can result from direct trauma to iliac crest or ASIS resulting in a contusion	■ TTP @ iliac crest/ASIS ■ Pain with resisted hip flexion & stretching into hip extension ■ Pain with ambulation & hip abduction ■ Screen for McBurney's point & rebound tenderness ■ (−) X-ray; need to r/o fx & avulsion
Labral Tear—damage to fibrocartilage via degeneration due to repetitive hip ER or the application of an external rotatory force to the hip while in hyperextension & hyperabduction; highly associated with hip dysplasia; anterior hip pain is correlated to weak gluteals & abdominals 2° excessive anterior femoral translation	■ Pain with prolonged sitting, getting in/out of a car, putting on shoes/socks, & twisting activities ■ ↑ Anterior hip pain with hyperext & ER ■ Pain with resisted SLR (anterior lesion) ■ Often associated with weak gluteals ■ ↓ Hip ROM; clicking/catching from flexion to extension ■ (+) Tests: FABER, impingement, Scour & labral tests ■ Screen for osteoid osteoma & testicular CA in ♂ ■ MRI with contrast is best dx test (is often inconclusive)

Continued

Pathology/Mechanism	Signs/Symptoms
Avulsion Fracture—injury results from violent muscle contraction	■ May hear a "pop" ■ Pain with stretch & contraction; TTP @ apophysis ■ (1) Tests: Thomas' & Ely's ■ May need CT or MRI if x-ray is inconclusive ■ Need to r/o strain & slipped capital femoral epiphysis
Femoral Neck Stress Fracture—gradual onset with history of endurance tasks **Beware** of eating disorders, amenorrhea, & osteoporosis	■ Groin pain with activity ■ TTP @ greater trochanter ■ (+) FABER test ■ May need CT or MRI if x-ray is inconclusive ■ Need to r/o trochanteric bursitis & osteoid osteoma
Degenerative Joint Disease—usually occurs >55 yo in ♀ > ♂ (3:2)	■ Aching pain during WB => groin, medial thigh & knee ■ Loss of movement & function ■ Trendelenburg ■ (+) FABER test ■ X-ray reveals narrow joint space, spurring & osteophytes; can r/o fx & necrosis
RA—systemic disorder with bilateral WB symptoms	■ Aching pain during WB => groin, medial thigh & distal knee; loss of movement & function 2° pain ■ Trendelenburg ■ (+) Tests: Thomas', Ely's & FABER ■ X-ray = bilateral demineralization of femoral head; joint space narrowing; migration of femoral head into acetabulum

Continued

Pathology/Mechanism	Signs/Symptoms
Slipped Capital Femoral Epiphysis imbalance of growth & hormones that weakens the epiphyseal plate; may be 2° ↑ wt gain; occurs in 10–16 yo ♂ 2x > ♀	■ Gradual onset of unilateral hip, thigh & knee pain ■ ↓ Hip IR; hip positioned in flexion, abd, ER ■ Quadriceps atrophy ■ Antalgic gait & ↓ limb length ■ AP x-ray needed to identify widening of physis & ↓ ht of epiphysis; lateral view = epiphyseal displacement ■ Need to r/o muscle strain & avulsion
Legg-Calvé-Perthes (LCPD) Disorder—idiopathic osteonecrosis of capital femoral epiphysis; associated with (+) family history & breech birth. Onset occurs over 1–3 months between 4–13 yo; occurs unilaterally; ♂ > ♀	■ Hip or groin pain (thigh resulting in antalgic gait ■ (+) Trendelenburg ■ ↓ ROM (ext, IR & abd); >15° hip flexion contracture ■ Leg length inequality; thigh atrophy ■ Bone scan or MRI needed for early detection, x-rays may appear normal for several weeks, 1st sign (~4 wks) is radiolucent crescent image parallel to the superior rim of the femoral head ■ Need to r/o JRA & hip inflammation
Osteoid osteoma—benign tumor found in long bones; etiology unknown	■ Vague hip pain @ night ■ ↑ Pain with activity & ↓ with aspirin ■ ↓ ROM & quad atrophy ■ May be apparent on x-ray but confirmed by MRI or CT ■ Need to r/o trochanteric bursitis, femoral neck stress fx
Myositis Ossificans—calcium deposits 2° contusion to the thigh	■ Localized pain ■ Limited knee flexion ■ Palpation of a calcific mass

Continued

Pathology/Mechanism	Signs/Symptoms
Hip Dislocation—may result from a breech birth, trauma, or when the hip is in a weakened state after a THR	■ (+) Tests: Ortolani's & Barlow's ■ (+) X-ray (associated with torticollis) ***Congenital*** ■ Shortened limb, positioned in flexion & abduction ***Posterior Traumatic (MVA)*** ■ Groin & lateral hip pain ■ Shortened limb, positioned in flexion, adduction & IR ***Anterior Traumatic (forced abduction)*** ■ Groin pain & tenderness ■ Positioned in extension & ER if superior/anterior ■ Positioned in flexion, abduction & ER if inferior/anterior

Knee Anatomy

Anterior

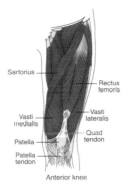

Sartorius

Rectus femoris

Vasti medialis

Vasti lateralis

Quad tendon

Patella

Patella tendon

Anterior knee

Posterior

Medial

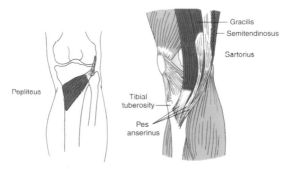

Popliteus

Gracilis

Semitendinosus

Sartorius

Tibial tuberosity

Pes anserinus

Medical Red Flags

- **Night pain** = tumor or infection
- **Cellulitis**
  - Recent hx of skin trauma
  - Pain, swelling, warmth
  - Advancing erythema with reddish streaks
  - Chills, fever, weakness
- **DVT risk**
  - Immobilization
  - Surgery
  - Fracture or trauma
  - Oral contraceptives
  - CHF, CA, DM
  - Pregnancy
- ***DVT Clinical presentation***
  - Leg pain & tenderness
  - ↑ Circumference > 1.2 cm
  - Tissue warm & firm to palpation
  - ↑ Pain with BP cuff inflated to 160 mm Hg
  - (+) Homans' sign

Imaging

Ottawa Knee Rule

X-ray series is only required if the patient presents with any of the following criteria:

- >55 years old
- Isolated tenderness of the patella
- Tenderness of the head of the fibula
- Inability to flex >90°
- Inability to bear weight (4 steps) *both* immediately after injury & in emergency department (regardless of limping)

Statistics: Adults: Sensitivity = 98%–100% & specificity = 19%–54%
Children: Sensitivity = 92% & specificity = 49%

Toolbox Tests

Western Ontario & McMaster Universities Osteoarthritis Index (WOMAC)

Instructions: Please rate the activities in each category according to the following scale of difficulty:

0 = none; 1 = slight; 2 = moderate; 3 = very; 4 = extremely

Pain		
	■ Walking	
	■ Stair climbing	
	■ Nocturnal	
	■ Rest	
	■ Weight bearing	
Stiffness	■ Morning stiffness	
	■ Stiffness occurring later in the day	
Physical Function	■ Descending stairs	
	■ Ascending stairs	
	■ Rising from sitting	
	■ Standing	
	■ Bending to floor	
	■ Walking on flat surface	
	■ Getting in/out of car	
	■ Going shopping	
	■ Putting on socks	
	■ Lying in bed	
	■ Taking off socks	
	■ Rising from bed	
	■ Getting in/out of bath	
	■ Sitting	
	■ Getting on/off toilet	
	■ Heavy domestic duties	
	■ Light domestic duties	
Total Score		

Scoring: Summate the scores of each item for the total score. The higher the score, the more severe the disability.

Source: From Bellamy, et al. Journal of Rheumatology, 15:1833–1840, 1988.

Lysholm Knee Rating System

Which items below best describe your knee function today?

Limp	None	5
	Slight or periodic	3
	Severe & constant	0
Support	None	5
	Cane or crutch needed	2
	Weight bearing impossible	0
Locking	None	15
	Catching sensation but no locking	10
	Locking occasionally	6
	Locking frequently	2
	Locked joint at examination	0
Instability	Never gives way	25
	Rarely during physical activity	20
	Frequently during physical activity	15
	Occasionally during daily activity	10
	Often during daily activity	5
	Every step	0
Pain	None	25
	Intermittent during strenuous activity	20
	Marked during strenuous activity	15
	Marked with walking >2 km (1.2 miles)	10
	Marked with walking <2 km (1.2 miles)	5
	Constant	0
Swelling	None	10
	After strenuous activities	6
	After ordinary activities	2
	Constant	0

Continued

Lysholm Knee Rating System—*cont'd*

Which items below best describe your knee function today?

Stairs	No problem	10
	Slight problem	6
	One step at a time	2
	Impossible	0
Squatting	No problem	5
	Slight problem	4
	Not >90° knee flexion (halfway)	2
	Impossible	0
Total Score		

Scoring: Summate the scores of each category. The higher the score, the greater the functional abilities.

Source: From Tegner, Y, Lysholm, J. Rating systems in the evaluation of knee ligament injuries. Clin Orthop Relat Res. 1985 Sep;(198):43–49.

Referral Patterns

Muscle Pain Referral Patterns

Rectus femoris

Vasti muscles

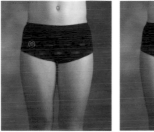 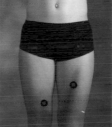

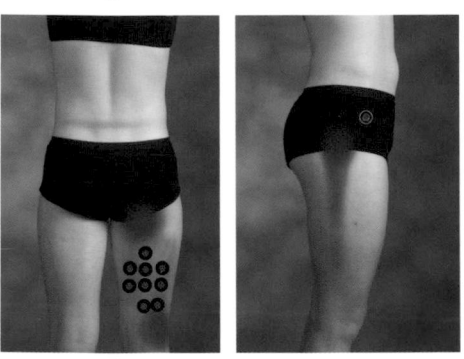

Hamstring muscles   Tensor fascia latae

Palpation Pearls

- **Adductor tubercle** = attachment of adductor magnus; start on medial femoral condyle & move proximal between the vastus medialis & hamstring tendons, as the femur dips in, a small point is palpable & often tender
- **Lateral collateral ligament** = cross leg so ankle is on contralateral knee (figure 4 position); LCL is palpable at the joint line just proximal to fibular head (firm, pencil-thickness structure)
- **Common peroneal nerve** = posterior lateral knee between biceps femoris tendon & lateral gastroc muscle belly
- **Popliteus** = "unlocker" of the knee; deep muscle only the tendon is palpable; follow the tibial tuberosity medially around the knee to the posterior aspect & the popliteus tendon is deep to the gastroc/soleus
- **Q-angle** = the angle created by the intersection of a line from the ASIS to the mid-patella & a line from the mid-patella to the tibial tuberosity. Normal (supine) = 13°–18° for ♀ & 10°–15° for ♂

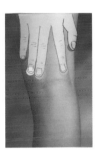

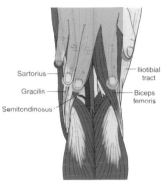

Strength & Function

- Concentric Quad to Hamstring ratio = 5:3 (i.e., hamstrings should be 60%–65% of quads)
- Quad:Hamstring ratio should approach 5:4 at the conclusion of ACL rehabilitation
- Quad:Hamstring ratio should approach 5:2 at the conclusion of PCL rehabilitation

Osteokinematics of the Knee

Normal ROM	OPP	CPP	Normal End-feel(s)	Abnormal End-feel(s)
Flexion >130° Rotation = 10°	25° flexion	Maximal extension & tibial ER	Flexion = tissue approximation Extension = elastic/firm SLR = elastic	Springy block = displaced meniscus Boggy = ligamentous pathology

- Femoral condyles begin to contact the patella inferior @ 20° of knee flexion; progresses superior @ 90° & medial/lateral @ 135° of knee flexion
- Structures attached to medial meniscus = MCL & semimembranosus
- Structures attached to lateral meniscus = PCL & popliteus

Arthrokinematics for Knee Mobilization

Concave surface: Tibial plateau Convex surface: Femoral condyles	To facilitate knee extension: OKC = Tibia rolls & glides anterior on the femur CKC = Femur rolls anterior & glides posterior on tibia	To facilitate knee flexion: OKC = Tibia rolls & glides posterior on the femur CKC = Femur rolls posterior & glides anterior on the tibia

Special Tests

LACHMAN'S TEST

Purpose: Assess for ACL laxity

Position: Supine with knee in 0-30° of flexion (hamstrings relaxed)

Technique: Stabilize distal femur & translate proximal tibia forward on the femur

Interpretation: + test = >5 mm of displacement or a mushy, soft end-feel; beware of false (–) test due to hamstring guarding, hemarthrosis, posterior medial meniscus tear

Statistics: Sensitivity = 63%–99% & specificity = 90%–99%

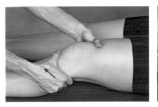 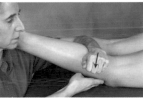

PRONE LACHMAN'S TEST

Purpose: Assess for ACL laxity

Position: Prone with knee flexed to 30°, LE supported & hamstrings relaxed

Technique: Palpate anterior aspect of the knee while imparting an anterior force to posterior-proximal aspect of tibia

Interpretation: + test = >5 mm of displacement or a mushy, soft end-feel

Beware of false (–) test due to hamstring guarding, hemarthrosis, posterior medial meniscus tear

ANTERIOR DRAWER TEST

Purpose: Assess for ACL laxity
Position: Supine with foot stabilized on table, knee flexed to 80°–90° & hamstrings relaxed

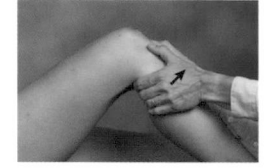

Technique: Translate proximal tibia anterior on the femur
Interpretation: + test = >5mm of anterior displacement; snap or palpable jerk with anterior drawer indicates meniscus px
Beware: Translation may appear excessive with PCL injury if tibia starts from a more posterior position
Statistics: Sensitivity = 22%–95% & specificity = 78%–97%

POSTERIOR DRAWER TEST

Purpose: Assess for PCL laxity
Position: Supine with knee flexed to 90° & foot on table

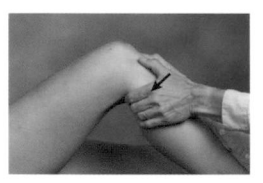

Technique: Translate proximal tibia posteriorly on distal femur
Interpretation: + test = >5 mm of posterior displacement
Statistics: Sensitivity = 86%–90% & specificity = 99%

SAG or GODFREY'S TEST

Purpose: Assess for PCL laxity
Position: Supine 90/90, support LEs
Technique: Compare the level of the tibial tuberosities

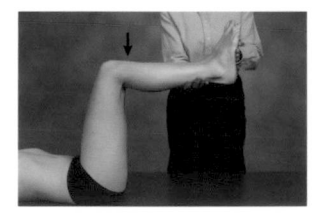

Interpretation: + test = posterior displacement of the tibial tuberosity is greater in the involved lag
Statistics: Sensitivity = 79% & specificity = 100%

CLARKE'S TEST; GRIND TEST; ZOHLER'S TEST

Purpose: Assess for chondromalacia or patella malacia

Position: Supine with knee in extension, clinician compresses quads at the superior pole of the patella to resist patella movement

Technique: Client contracts quads against resistance

Interpretation: + test = inability to contract without pain

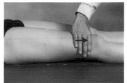

VARUS TEST

Purpose: Assess for LCL laxity

Position: Supine; knee in full extension & then repeat @ 30° flexion

Technique: Cup knee with heel of clinician's hand @ medial joint line; use fingers of other hand to palpate lateral joint line; apply a varus stress to the knee through the palm of the medial hand & the forearm/elbow of the lateral hand

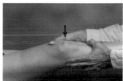

Interpretation: + test = pain or excessive gapping of the joint when compared with the contralateral side

Statistics: Sensitivity = 25%

VALGUS TEST

Purpose: Assess for MCL laxity

Position: Supine; knee in full extension & then repeat @ 30° flexion

Technique: Cup knee with heel of clinician's hand @ lateral joint line; use fingers of other hand to palpate medial joint line; apply a valgus stress to the knee through the palm of the lateral hand & the forearm/elbow of the medial hand

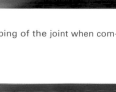

Interpretation: + test = pain or excessive gapping of the joint when compared to the contralateral side

Statistics: Sensitivity = 86%–96%

APLEY'S TEST

Purpose: Assess meniscus (nonspecific for location of meniscal tear)

Position: Prone, knee flexed to 90°; clinician grasps foot & calcaneus

Technique: While applying a downward force through the heel, rotate the tibia internally & externally

Interpretation: + test = pain, popping, snapping, locking, crepitus

Statistics: Sensitivity = 13%–58% & specificity = 80%–93%

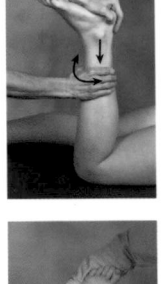

McMURRAY'S TEST

Purpose: Assess meniscus

Position: Supine, with 1 of clinician's hands to the side of the patella & the other grasping the distal tibia

Technique: From a position of maximal flexion, extend the knee with IR of the tibia & a varus stress then returns to maximal flexion & extend the knee with ER of the tibia & a valgus stress

Interpretation: + test = pain or snapping/clicking with IR incriminates the lateral meniscus & ER incriminates the medial meniscus; if pain, snapping, or clicking occur with the knee in flexion, the posterior horn of the meniscus is involved & if the pain, snapping, or clicking occurs with increasing amounts of knee extension, the anterior meniscus is involved

Statistics: Sensitivity = 16%–67% & specificity = 57%–98%

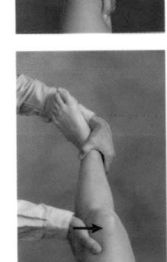

THESSALY'S TEST

Purpose: Assess for meniscal tears

Position: Standing on the involved LE with the knee flexed @ 5°

Technique: Clinician holds pt's outstretched arms & rotates internally then externally 3x; repeat @ 20° of knee flexion

Interpretation: + test = Pt experiences locking or catching

Statistics: At 5°: Sensitivity = 66%–81% & specificity = 91%–96% and at 20°: Sensitivity = 89%–92% & specificity = 96%–97%

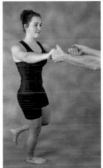

PATELLA APPREHENSION (FAIRBANK'S) TEST

Purpose: Assess for subluxing patella

Position: Supine or seated, 30° knee flexion, quads relaxed

Technique: Clinician carefully pushes patella laterally

Interpretation: + test = Pt feels patella about to dislocate & contracts quads to keep this from happening

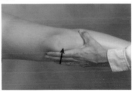

Statistics: Sensitivity = 32%–39% & specificity = 86%

PATELLA TILT TEST

Purpose: Assess for ITB tightness/patella mobility

Position: Relaxed in supine with knee in extension

Technique: Clinician attempts to lift the lateral border of patella

Interpretation: + test = inability to lift the lateral border of the patella above the horizontal

NOBLE'S TEST

Purpose: Assess ITB irritation
Position: Supine, start @ 90/90
Technique: Apply pressure over the lateral femoral condyle while extending the knee
Interpretation: + test = pain or clicking @ lateral femoral condyle @ 30° of knee flexion

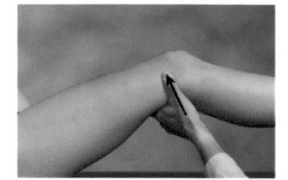

OBER'S TEST

Purpose: Assess for tight ITB
Position: Side-lying with involved hip up
Technique: Extend the hip & allow LE to drop into adduction
Interpretation: + test = LE fails to adduct past anatomic neutral

RENNE'S TEST

Purpose: Assess ITB irritation
Position: Standing
Technique: Apply pressure over the lateral femoral condyle with AROM of the knee
Interpretation: + test = pain or clicking @ lateral femoral condyle @ 30° of knee flexion

PIVOT SHIFT TEST
Purpose: Assess A/L instability
Position: Supine
Technique: Knee is taken from full extension to flexion with a valgus stress
Interpretation: + test = sudden reduction of the anteriorly subluxed lateral tibial plateau

STUTTER TEST
Purpose: Assess for medial plica irritation
Position: Sitting with knee flexed over the edge of the table
Technique: Slowly extend knee with a finger placed lightly in contact with the center of the patella
Interpretation: + test = patella stutters as knee moves into extension

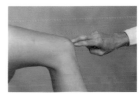

PATELLAR BOWSTRING TEST
Purpose: Assess medial plica
Position: Supine
Technique: Medially displace patella while flexing/extending knee with tibia IR
Interpretation: + test = palpable clunk

WILSON'S TEST
Purpose: Assess for osteochondritis of medial femoral condyle
Position: Supine with knee flexed to 90°
Technique: Extend the knee with IR of the tibia
Interpretation: + test = pain at 30° of flexion in IR that ↓ if the tibia is ER; should r/o meniscal px

Pathology/Mechanism	Signs/Symptoms
Baker's Cyst—defect in the posterior capsule that is influenced by chronic irritation	■ Golf ball–size swelling at semi-membranosus tendon or medial gastroc muscle belly; best palpated in full knee extension ■ Stiff & tender with limited knee ROM ■ MRI may be helpful; need to r/o DVT & tumor
Shin Splints/Anterior—an overuse syndrome of tibialis anterior, extensor hallicus longus, & extensor digitorum longus attributed to running on unconditioned legs, soft tissue imbalance, alignment abnormalities, & excessive pronation to accommodate rearfoot varus	■ Pain & tenderness over anterior tibialis ■ Pain with resisted dorsiflexion & inversion ■ Pain with stretching into plantarflexion & eversion ■ Callus formation under 2nd metatarsal head & medial side of distal hallux ■ Tight gastroc/soleus ■ Soreness with heel walking ■ (–) X-ray, needed to r/o stress fx
Shin Splints/Posterior—an overuse syndrome of flexor hallucis longus & flexor digitorum longus; rapid & excessive pronation to compensate for rearfoot varus; result is ↑ stress on tibialis posterior to decelerate pronation	■ Callus formation under 2nd> 3rd> 4th MT head & medial side of distal hallux ■ Pain & soreness over distal 1/3–2/3 of posterior/medial shin & posterior medial malleolus ■ Hypermobile 1st MTP ■ Pain with resisted inversion & plantarflexion ■ Pain with stretching into dorsiflexion & eversion ■ (–) X-ray, needed to r/o stress fx

Continued

Pathology/Mechanism	Signs/Symptoms
Compartment Syndrome—a progression of shin splints resulting in a loss of microcirculation in shin muscle; ♂ > ♀, R > L **Beware:** This is an emergency situation	■ ↑ Soft tissue pressures via fluid accumulation ■ Ischemia of extensor hallicus longus ■ Skin feels warm & firm ■ Pain with stretch or AROM; foot drop ■ Most reliable sign is sensory deficit of the dorsum of foot in 1st interdigital cleft ■ Pulses are normal until the end & then surgery within 4–6 hours is required to prevent muscle necrosis & nerve damage ■ Confirmed with MRI & pressure assessment
Bursitis—mechanical irritation ■ prepatella = common in sport = falling on knee or maintaining quadruped position (housemaids knee) ■ infrapatella = clergyman bursitis = kneeling (mechanical irritation) ■ pes anserine = prevalent in long-distance running or middle-aged females with OA of the knee	■ Localized radiating heat ■ Localized egg-shaped swelling ■ Radiating pain 2–4 cm below the involved bursa ■ Crepitus ■ Discomfort with A & PROM ■ Diagnosis confirmed with MRI
Popliteus Tendonitis—results from overuse, downhill running, activities with sudden stops	■ Posterior lateral knee pain at the end of a workout or running downhill (just posterior to LCL) ■ Crepitus over tendon ■ Discomfort sitting with legs crossed & initiating flexion against resistance from full extension ■ MRI may be helpful; need to r/o ITB, biceps tendonitis

Continued

Pathology/Mechanism	Signs/Symptoms
Jumper's Knee = patella tendonitis (most common in skeletally immature) 2° traction overuse injury such as jumping, kicking, running or degenerative process 2° microtrauma	■ TTP at patella tendon insertion & pain with resisted knee extension ■ Localized crepitus & swelling ■ ↑ Q-angle ■ Need to r/o Osgood-Schlatter's, SLJ, & bursitis ■ Confirmed with MRI
ITB Friction Syndrome—repetitive stress & excessive friction 2° tight ITB, pronation with IR of tibia, genu varum, cycling with cleat in IR Proximal px = hip syndrome Distal px = runner's knee	■ Pain with downhill running ■ Pain @ 30° of knee flexion in WB results in ambulating stiff legged to avoid flexion ■ TTP over lateral femoral condyle ■ (+) Tests: Ober's, Noble's, & Renne's ■ (–) X-ray ■ Need to r/o trochanteric bursitis & osteochondritis ■ MRI & US may confirm diagnosis
Plica Syndrome—injury results from direct trauma or a significant ↑ in unaccustomed activity (presence of medial plica is more common than a lateral plica)	■ Pain over medial femoral condyle; palpable cords along medial condyle, pain at superomedial joint line ■ Reports of clicking/snapping, locking, "giving way" ■ Full ROM but pain at end range flexion ■ False (+) McMurray (pseudolocking) ■ (+) Tests: Stutter, plica, theatre sign & bowstring ■ Need to r/o patellofemoral tracking px ■ X-ray is not helpful, MRI is only noninvasive procedure that shows plica ■ Arthroscope may reveal an avascular fibrotic edge of the plica

Continued

Pathology/Mechanism	Signs/Symptoms
Chondromalacia (patellofemoral syndrome–PFS)—softening of the patella articular cartilage 2° poor biomechanical alignment/tracking &/or weak hip ER	■ Anterior knee pain; pain with stairs; crepitus ■ VMO atrophy; weak hip ER ■ ↑ Knee valgus, ↑ Q-angle ■ (+) Tests: Theater, Clarke's, & Fairbank's/apprehension ■ Confirmed via MRI
Patella Subluxation—predisposing factors include excessive tibial ER, pronation, patella alta, tight lateral retinaculum, weak hip ER, small medial patella facet; most common in adolescent girls with genu valgum (↑ Q-angle & femoral rotation)	■ Effusion shuts down VMO ■ (+) Tests: Patella tilt & patella apprehension ■ Tenderness along medial patella border ■ Sitting @ 90/90, patella points lateral & superior (grasshopper eyes) ■ Client c/o knee giving way or clicking when cutting away from affected leg ■ ↑ Q-angle ■ X-ray may reveal osteochondral fragments or fx; multiple views are needed to evaluate all articular surfaces
Patella Fracture—results from direct trauma	■ Pain & "dome" effusion; palpable defect ■ Unable to extend knee ■ Confirmed with x-ray
LCL Sprain—injury results from varus stress resulting in over-stretching or tearing of the LCL	■ Warm & swollen lateral knee ■ TTP @ knee joint line (palpate in figure-4 position) ■ ROM may not be effected ■ (+) Varus stress test ■ Confirmed with MRI or arthrogram with contrast ■ (–) X-ray but needed to r/o avulsion or epiphyseal plate injury; Varus stress film may show ↑ joint gapping

Continued

Pathology/Mechanism	Signs/Symptoms
MCL Sprain—injury results from valgus stress resulting in over-stretching or tearing of the MCL	■ Flexion limited to 90° & knee extension lag present ■ If deep fibers are torn, knee joint rapidly fills with blood ■ (+) Valgus stress test ■ TTP @ knee joint line (possible palpable defect) ■ Confirmed with MRI or arthrogram with contrast ■ (–) X-ray but needed to r/o avulsion or epiphyseal plate injury; valgus stress film may show ↑ joint gapping
ACL Sprain—injury results from twisting while changing directions, deceleration with valgus & ER, hyperflexion of the knee with foot in plantarflexion	■ Audible pop with immediate swelling (<2 hrs) ■ Intense pain at posterior lateral tibia ■ Unstable in WB ■ (+) Tests: Anterior drawer, Lachman's, & pivot shift ■ KT1000/2000 anterior displacement >5 mm ■ (–) X-ray (except for avulsion); MRI is study of choice ■ Bloody arthrocentesis
PCL Sprain—injury results from dashboard blow to anterior shin with knee flexed @ 90° or falling on the knee with foot plantarflexed	■ Minimal swelling; ecchymosis may appear days later ■ Tenderness in popliteal fossa & pain with kneeling ■ Pt may be able to continue to play ■ (+) Tests: Posterior drawer, posterior Lachman's, & SAG/dropback/Godfrey's ■ (–) X-ray (except for avulsion); MRI is study of choice ■ Bloody arthrocentesis

Continued

Pathology/Mechanism	Signs/Symptoms
Meniscus Tear—injured via rotatory forces while WB or hyperextension of knee; medial femoral/lateral tibial rotation injures medial meniscus & lateral femoral/medial tibial rotation injures lateral meniscus. *Common types of tears:* Children = longitudinal & peripheral tear Teenagers = bucket handle tear	■ (−) Varus/valgus stress ■ Pain at end range flexion/extension & WB ■ Gradual swelling over 1-3 days; ecchymosis ■ Joint line tenderness ■ (+) Tests: McMurray's & Apley's (unreliable in children) ■ Anterior horn locks in extension, posterior in flexion, medial in 10°–30° of flexion, lateral >70° of flexion ■ X-ray may r/o fx, tumor, osseous loose bodies ■ MRI may reveal pseudotear; confirm with arthrogram using contrast
DJD—result of aging, poor biomechanics or repetitive trauma	■ Joint line crepitus ■ ↓ Terminal knee extension 2° to edema (quad atrophy) ■ ↓ Stance time during gait ■ "Gelling" phenomenon = ↑ viscosity of synovial fluid 2° to inflammation ■ Anteriomedial knee pain & stiffness with immobility ■ X-ray will reveal narrow joint space, spurring, osteophytes
Osgood-Schlatter's Disease—tibial apophysitis that may occur from rapid growth of femur resulting in avulsion of proximal tibial physis; may have a genetic predisposition; 8–15 yo, ♂ > ♀	■ Intermittent aching pain at tibial tubercle & distal patellar tendon ■ Enlarged tibial tuberosity ■ Tight quads & hamstrings resulting in ↓ AROM ■ Effusion results in knee extensor lag ■ (+) Ely test ■ (+) X-ray for avulsion of tibial tuberosity (lateral view) ■ Need to r/o avascular necrosis

Continued

Pathology/Mechanism	Signs/Symptoms
Sinding-Larsen Johansson (SLJ)—results from a traction force on the patella tendon 2° chronic extensor overload; 10–14 yo ♂	■ Anterior knee pain & TTP at distal pole of the patella with knee extension ■ Antalgic gait ■ ↓ Knee ROM ■ X-ray (lateral view)= fragmentation of inferior patella pole
Myositis Ossificans—calcification in a muscle due to trauma, painful hematoma develop rapidly & calcification occurs in 2–3 wks; ossification occurs in 4–8 wks; may be neurogenic after a SCI or TBI	■ Warm & TTP over involved site ■ ↓ ROM ■ Pain with contraction of involved muscle ■ Confirmed with x-ray after 2–3 weeks; earlier with MRI
Heterotropic Ossification—ossification between rather than within strained muscle fibers resulting from direct trauma	■ ↓ ROM ■ Weakness of involved muscle ■ TTP, swelling, & hyperemia ■ Confirmed with x-ray after 2–3 weeks; earlier with MRI
Osteochondritis Dissecans—lesions of subchondral bone of insidious onset; possible trauma vs preexisting abnormalities of epiphyses; most common in posterolateral medial femoral condyle; 10–18 yo; ♂ > ♀	■ Knee effusion ■ Crepitus with knee flexion/extension & effusion ■ Poorly localized knee pain ■ Antalgic gait ■ (+) Wilson's test ■ May have TTP over medial femoral condyle with knee flexion ■ X-ray may not help; need MRI or bone scan

Ankle & Foot Anatomy

Medial view of ankle ligaments

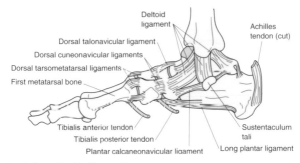

Deltoid ligament

Achilles tendon (cut)

Dorsal talonavicular ligament

Dorsal cuneonavicular ligaments

Dorsal tarsometatarsal ligaments

First metatarsal bone

Tibialis anterior tendon

Tibialis posterior tendon

Plantar calcaneonavicular ligament

Sustentaculum tali

Long plantar ligament

Lateral view of ankle ligaments

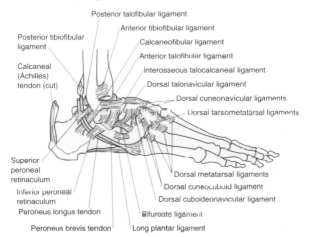

Posterior talofibular ligament

Anterior tibiofibular ligament

Calcaneofibular ligament

Anterior talofibular ligament

Interosseous talocalcaneal ligament

Dorsal talonavicular ligament

Posterior tibiofibular ligament

Calcaneal (Achilles) tendon (cut)

Dorsal cuneonavicular ligaments

Dorsal tarsometatarsal ligaments

Superior peroneal retinaculum

Inferior peroneal retinaculum

Peroneus longus tendon

Peroneus brevis tendon

Dorsal metatarsal ligaments

Dorsal cuneocuboid ligament

Dorsal cuboideonavicular ligament

Bifurcate ligament

Long plantar ligament

Medical Red Flags

- **Paresthesia**—stocking distribution, associated with:
  - DM
  - Lead/mercury poison
- **Gout**
  - Swelling & TTP @ 1st MTP or ankle
  - Pain with A & PROM of foot &/or ankle
  - Hypersensitive to touch
- **Lyme's Disease**
  - "Bull's eye" rash (expanding red rings)
  - Flu-like symptoms
- **Bilateral ankle edema** with ↑ BP with hx of NSAIDS use may be the result of renal vasoconstriction

Complex Regional Pain Syndrome

Stage 1	■ Burning, aching, tenderness, joint stiffness ■ Swelling, temperature changes ■ ↑ nail growth & ↑ hair on foot/feet
Stage 2	■ ↑ Pain, swelling, joint stiffness ■ Pain becomes less localized ■ Change in skin color & texture
Stage 3	■ Pain radiates all the way up the leg ■ ↓ Nerve conduction velocity ■ Muscle atrophy

Imaging

Ottawa Ankle Rules

Radiographic series of the *ankle* is only required if one of the following are present:

- Bone tenderness at posterior edge of the distal 6 cm of the medial malleolus
- Bone tenderness at posterior edge of the distal 6 cm of the lateral malleolus
- Totally unable to bear weight *both* immediately after injury & (for 4 steps) in the emergency department

Statistics: Adults: Sensitivity = 95%–100% & specificity = 16%
Children: Sensitivity = 83%–100% & specificity = 21%–50%

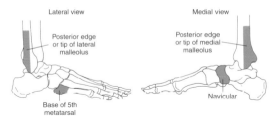

Lateral view

Posterior edge or tip of lateral malleolus

Base of 5th metatarsal

Medial view

Posterior edge or tip of medial malleolus

Navicular

Ottawa Foot Rules

Radiographic series of the *foot* is only required if one of the following are present:

- Bone tenderness is at navicular
- Bone tenderness at the base of 5th MT
- Totally unable to bear weight *both* immediately after injury & (for 4 steps) in the emergency department

Statistics: Adults: Sensitivity = 93-100% & specificity = 12-21%
Children: Sensitivity = 100% & specificity = 36%

A Performance Test Protocol and Scoring Scale for the Evaluation of Ankle Injuries

Subjective Assessment of the Injured Ankle		Can You Walk Normally?	
No symptoms	15	Yes	15
Mild symptoms	10		
Moderate symptoms	5	No	0
Severe symptoms	0		

Can You Run Normally?		Climb Down Stairs? (2 flights ~ 44 steps)	
Yes	15	Under 18 seconds	10
No	0	18-20 seconds	5
		>20 seconds	0

Rising on Heels with Injured Leg		Rising on Toes with Injured Leg	
>40 seconds	10	>40 seconds	10
30-39 seconds	5	30-39 seconds	5
<30 seconds	0	<30 seconds	0

Single-limbed Stance with Injured Leg		Laxity of Ankle Joints	
>55 seconds	10	Stable (5 mm)	10
50-54 seconds	5	Moderate laxity (6-10 mm)	5
>50 seconds	0	Severe laxity (>10 mm)	0

Injured Leg Dorsiflexion ROM		TOTAL SCORE:	
≥10°	10		
5-9°	5		
<5°	0		

Scoring: Summate all scores

Excellent = 85-100; Good = 70-80; Fair = 55-65; Poor ≤50

Source: From American Journal of Sports Medicine, 22(4):462-9, 1994 Jul-Aug.

Foot Function Index

Mark the horizontal lines below to address each task.

How severe is your foot pain?

No pain   Worse pain
                                                           imaginable

At its worst

In the morning

Walking barefoot

Standing barefoot

Walking with shoes

Standing with shoes

Walking in orthotics

Standing in orthotics

End of the day

How much difficulty do you have:

No difficulty   So difficult
                                                           unable to

Walking in house

Walking outside

Walking 4 blocks

Climbing stairs

Continued

Foot Function Index—cont'd

How much difficulty do you have:	No difficulty								So difficult unable to
Descending stairs									
Standing tip toe									
Getting out of a chair									
Climbing curbs									
Walking fast									
Because of your feet, how much of the time do you:	None								All
Stay inside all day									
Stay in bed all day									
Limit activities									
Use assistive device indoors									
Use assistive device outdoors									

Total Score:

Scoring: Summate all scores, exclude items that are not applicable & multiple by 100.
The higher the number is, the greater the impairment.

Source: From Journal of Clinical Epidemiology, 44(6):561–570, 1991.

Referral Patterns

Muscle Pain Referral Patterns

Peroneus longus & brevis   Peroneus (Fibularis) tertius

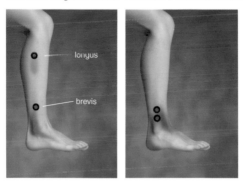

Tibialis anterior

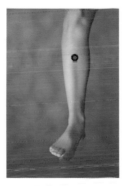

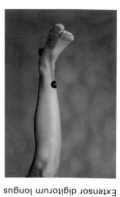

Extensor digitorum longus

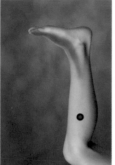

Extensor hallucis longus

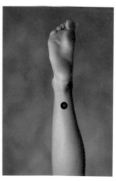

Flexor hallucis longus

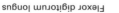

Flexor digitorum longus

Visual Inspection

- Hammer toe = hyperextension of MTP & DIP with PIP flexion of toes 2, 3, 4, 5; associated with hallux valgus; pain is worse with shoes on; corns present
- Hallux valgus = 1st MTP >20° valgus angle; 1st & 2nd toe overlap
- Index plus foot = 1st MT > 2nd > 3 > 4 > 5
- Index plus-minus foot = 1st MT = 2nd MT > 3 > 4 > 5
- Index minus foot = 1st MT < 2nd > 3 > 4 > 5
- Subtalar neutral = In the prone position with the forefoot passively dorsiflexed & pronated, it is the position in which the head of the talus is felt to be equally spaced from the navicular

Palpation Pearls

- *Dorsalis pedis artery* = on top of foot between 1st & 2nd metatarsals
- *Sustentaculum tali* = small ledge just distal to medial malleolus
- *Peroneal tubercle* = small prominence ~1" distal to lateral malleolus
- *Plantaris* = with knee flexed, palpate medial to posterior aspect of the fibula head, roll over lateral gastroc head and move slightly proximal; palpate for a 1"-wide muscle that runs on an angle from proximal/lateral to distal/medial
- *Tibialis anterior* = follow down the lateral tibial shaft to the medial aspect of the medial cuneiform
- *Extensor digitorum longus* = while extending the toes, follow the 4 prominent tendons proximal to the ankle—the tendons dive under the extensor retinaculum and emerge proximally as a thicker mass— follow the muscle belly along the tibia between the tibialis anterior and the peroneals (fibularis)

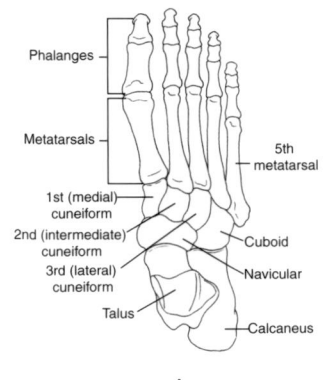

Superior view

Phalanges

Metatarsals

5th metatarsal

1st (medial) cuneiform

2nd (intermediate) cuneiform

Cuboid

3rd (lateral) cuneiform

Navicular

Talus

Calcaneus

A

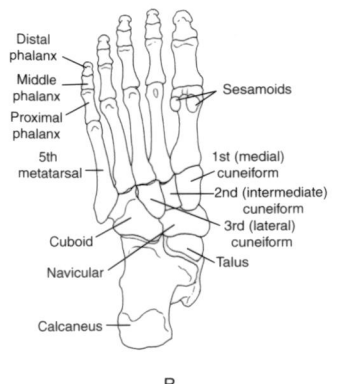

Inferior view

Distal phalanx

Middle phalanx

Proximal phalanx

Sesamoids

5th metatarsal

1st (medial) cuneiform

2nd (intermediate) cuneiform

3rd (lateral) cuneiform

Cuboid

Talus

Navicular

Calcaneus

B

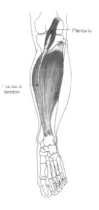

231
Extensor digitorum & ext hallucis

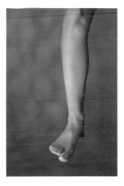

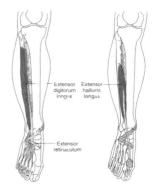

Extensor digitorum longus

Extensor hallucis longus

Extensor retinaculum

Plantaris

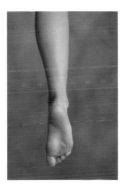

Plantaris

Plantaris tendon

Medial ankle structures

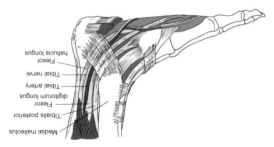

- Flexor hallucis longus
- Tibial nerve
- Tibial artery
- Flexor digitorum longus
- Tibialis posterior
- Medial malleolus

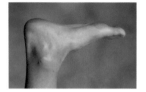

Lateral ankle structures

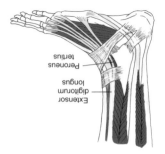

- Peroneus tertius
- Extensor digitorum longus

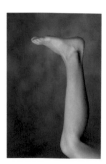

Plantar surface of the foot

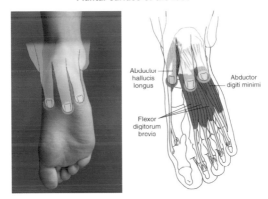

Abductor hallucis longus

Abductor digiti minimi

Flexor digitorum brevis

Feiss Line

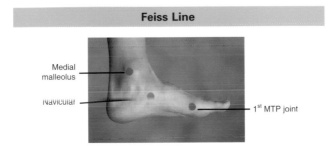

Medial malleolus

Navicular

1st MTP joint

In NWB, a line is constructed to connect the apex of the medial malleolus to the head of the 1st MTP joint. The navicular bone should be in line with these 2 structures. In the standing (WB) position, the navicular should not drop more than 2/3 the distance to the floor.

Girth Assessment

Figure-8 Method to Assess Ankle Edema

1. Start distal to the lateral malleolus; go medial, just distal to navicular tuberosity

2. Under the arch to the proximal aspect of the head of the 5th metatarsal

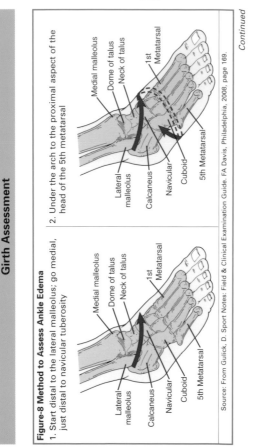

Medial malleolus
Dome of talus
Neck of talus
1st Metatarsal
Lateral malleolus
Calcaneus
Navicular
Cuboid
5th Metatarsal

Source: From Gulick, D. Sport Notes: Field & Clinical Examination Guide. FA Davis, Philadelphia, 2008, page 169.

Continued

235

Figure–8 Method to Assess Ankle Edema—cont'd

3. Across the anterior tibialis tendon to the distal aspect of the medial malleolus

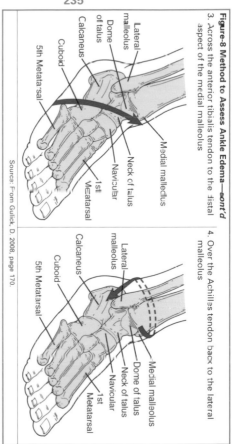

4. Over the Achilles tendon back to the lateral malleolus

Source: From Gulick, D. 2008, page 170.

Osteokinematics of the Ankle & Foot

Normal ROM		OPP	CPP	Normal End-feel(s)	Abnormal End-feel(s)
Plantarflexion 30°–50° Dorsiflexion 20° Inversion 10°–30° Eversion 10°–20°		10° PF	Maximal DF	Elastic (tissue stretch) for all planes	Empty = sprain/ strain
1st MTP	Extension 35°	5°–10° extension	Maximal extension	Capsular	Capsular = extension limited
2-5 MTP	Flexion 75°	Slight flexion	Maximal extension	Flex/extension = capsular/elastic Abd/adduction = ligamentous	Capsular = flexion limited

Arthrokinematics for Ankle & Foot Mobilization

Ankle flexion & extension	Concave surface: Distal tibia/fibula Convex surface: Talus	*To facilitate ankle dorsiflexion:* **OKC**—talus rolls anterior & glides posterior on tibia **CKC**—tibia rolls & glides anterior	*To facilitate ankle plantarflexion:* **OKC**—talus rolls posterior & glides anterior on tibia **CKC**—tibia rolls & glides posterior
Ankle inversion & eversion	Concave surface: Anterior calcaneal facet & posterior talus Convex surface: Posterior calcaneal facet & anterior talus	*To facilitate inversion:* **OKC**—anterior calcaneal facet rolls & glides medial while posterior calcaneal facet rolls & glides lateral **CKC**—talus rolls medial & glides lateral on anterior calcaneal facet while talus rolls & glides medial on posterior calcaneal facet	*To facilitate eversion:* **OKC**—anterior calcaneal facet rolls & glides lateral while posterior calcaneal facet rolls & glides medial **CKC**—talus rolls lateral & glides medial on anterior calcaneal facet while talus rolls & glides lateral on posterior calcaneal facet
MTP flexion & extension	Concave surface: Phalanx Convex surface: Metatarsal	*To facilitate flexion:* Phalanx rolls & glides distal/inferior on metatarsal	*To facilitate extension:* Phalanx rolls & glides proximal/superior on metatarsal

ANTERIOR DRAWER

Purpose: Assess for ATF laxity
Position: NWB position in ~ 20° of plantarflexion, stabilize the distal tibia/fibula
Technique: Grasp the posterior aspect of the calcaneus/talus & translate the calcaneus/talus anterior on the tibia/fibula
Interpretation: + test = pain & excessive movement 2° to instability

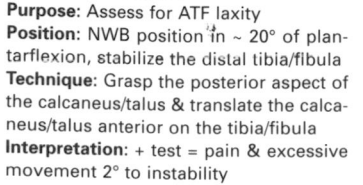

TALAR TILT

Purpose: Test for laxity of lateral ankle ligaments—ATF, CF, PTF
Position: NWB—stabilize the lower leg & palpate respective ligament
Technique: Grasp calcaneus to apply a varus stress to displace the talus from the mortise. Should be performed in plantarflexion (ATF), neutral (CF), & dorsiflexion (PTF)

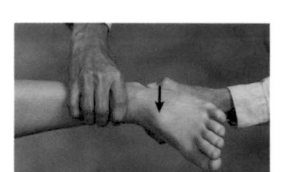

Interpretation: + test = pain or excessive gapping with respect to the contralateral limb

SQUEEZE TEST

Purpose: Assess for syndesmotic sprain
Position: Supine with knee extended
Technique: Begin at the proximal tibia/fibula & firmly compress (squeeze) the tibia/fibula together, progress distally toward the ankle until pain is elicited
Interpretation: + test = pain at the syndesmosis; the farther from the ankle the pain is elicited, the more severe the sprain

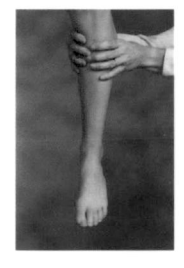

Note: Recovery time = 5 + (0.97 × cm from ankle joint that squeeze test is positive) ± 3 days

---

ER STRESS TEST (rotate from heel)
KLEIGER'S TEST (rotate from forefoot)

Purpose: Assess for deltoid or syndesmotic sprain

Position: Sitting with lower leg stabilized but syndesmosis not compressed

Technique: Grasp the heel or medial aspect of the foot & ER in plantarflexion (deltoid lig) & then repeat with ER in dorsiflexion (syndesmosis)

Interpretation: + test = pain or gapping as compared to contralateral limb

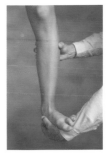

WINDLASS TEST

Purpose: Assess for plantar fasciitis

Position 1: NWB with knee flexed to 90°

Technique 1: Stabilize the ankle in neutral & dorsiflex the great toe

Interpretation 1: + test = pain along the medial longitudinal arch

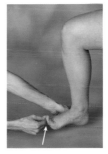

Position 2: WB

Technique 2: Standing on a stool with equal weight on both foot & toes hanging over the edge of the stool & dorsiflex the great toe

Interpretation 2: + test = pain along the medial longitudinal arch

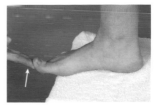

PERONEAL TENDON DISLOCATION

Purpose: Assess for damage to peroneal retinaculum
Position: Prone, knee flexed to 90°
Technique: Have the client actively plantarflex & dorsiflex the ankle against resistance
Interpretation: + test = tendon subluxing from behind the lateral malleolus

THOMPSON'S TEST

Purpose: Assess for Achilles tendon rupture
Position: Prone
Technique: Passively flex the knee to 90° & squeeze the middle 1/3 of the calf
Interpretation: Plantarflexion of the foot should occur; + test = failure to plantarflex

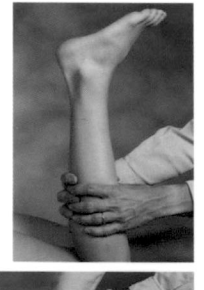

HOMAN'S SIGN

Purpose: Assess for thrombophlebitis of the lower leg
Position: Supine
Technique: Passively dorsiflex the foot & squeeze the calf
Interpretation: + test = sudden pain in the posterior leg or calf

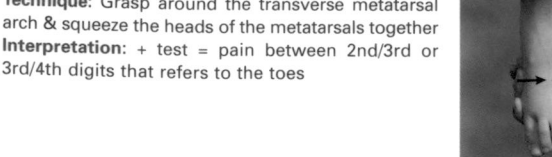

MORTON'S TEST

Purpose: Assess for neuroma
Position: NWB
Technique: Grasp around the transverse metatarsal arch & squeeze the heads of the metatarsals together
Interpretation: + test = pain between 2nd/3rd or 3rd/4th digits that refers to the toes

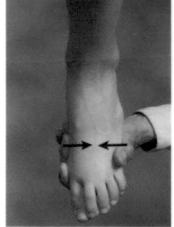

BUMP TEST

Purpose: Test for stress fx
Position: NWB—ankle in neutral
Technique: Apply a firm force with the thenar eminence to the heel of the foot
Interpretation: + test = pain at the site of the possible fx

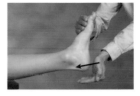

METATARSAL LOAD

Purpose: Assess for metatarsal fracture
Position: NWB
Technique: Grasp the distal aspect of the metatarsal bone & apply a longitudinal force to load the metatarsal
Interpretation: + test – localized pain as the metatarsal joints are compressed

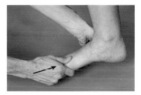

TINEL'S TEST

Purpose: Assess for tibial nerve damage
Position: NWB
Technique: Tap over posterior tibial nn (medial plantar nerve), just inferior & posterior to medial malleolus
Interpretation: + test = paresthesia into the foot

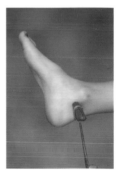

Pathology/Mechanism	Signs/Symptoms
Turf Toe—extreme hyperextension of great toe in CKC position resulting in sprain of plantar capsule & LCL of 1st MTP	■ Pain with toe extension ■ Impairment of push-off, antalgic gait ■ Ecchymosis & swelling of 1st MTP joint ■ (–) X-ray ■ Need to r/o sesamoid & metatarsal head fx
Hallux Valgus (Bunion)—RA, poor fitting footwear, flat feet	■ Pain, swelling, great toe valgus >15° ■ ↓ ROM of great toe & hammer 2nd toe ■ X-ray helpful ■ Need to r/o RA
Sesamoiditis—repetitive high impact sports or direct trauma	■ Impairment of push-off, antalgic gait, swollen 1st MTP ■ TTP, pain with passive dorsiflexion of MTP ■ (+) X-ray & MRI ■ Need to r/o turf toe & bipartite sesamoid
Stress Fracture—repetitive stresses occurs ~3 wks after ↑ training; (2nd MT is most common) **Beware** of eating disorders with repetitive stress fx	■ Deep nagging & localized pain; night pain ■ ROM WNL ■ (+) Tests: Metatarsal load & bump ■ Bone scan & MRI will detect earlier than x-ray ■ Therapeutic US in continuous mode will ↑ pain & may aid in dx ■ Need to r/o DVT
Hallux Rigidus—may be associated with osteochondritis (child) or DJD, gout, or RA (adult)	■ ↓ Dorsiflexion of 1st MTP joint ■ Pain & swelling on dorsal aspect of 1st MTP ■ Difficulty walking up stairs & uphill ■ ER of foot to clear LE during gait ■ X-ray will confirm dorsal osteophyte & ↓ joint space

Continued

Pathology/Mechanism	Signs/Symptoms
Charcot Foot—hypertrophic osteoarthropathy of midfoot in client's with IDDM	■ Progressive bone & muscle weakness ■ ↓ Sensation but minimal to no pain ■ Profound unilateral swelling ■ ↑ Skin temp (local); erythema ■ X-ray looks like osteomyelitis (bone fragments present)
Morton's Neuroma—thickening of interdigital nn (25–50 yo; ♀ > ♂) 2° high heel shoes, excessive pronation, high arch, lateral compression of forefoot, ↑ wt	■ Throbbing/burning into plantar aspect of 3rd & 4th MT heads; feels like a pebble is in the shoe ■ Callus under involved rays ■ ↑ Pain with WB, (+) Morton's test ■ Weak intrinsic muscles ■ EMG = unreliable ■ Need to r/o stress fx (MRI with contrast)
Plantarfascitis—continuous with gastroc mm; subject to inflammation 2° repetitive stress, poorly cushioned footwear, hard surfaces, ↑ pronation, obesity	■ Morning pain that ↓ with activity, nodules are palpable over proximal-medial border of plantar fascia ■ Pain with dorsiflexion & toe extension ■ ↓ Dorsiflexion due to tight gastroc ■ Weak foot intrinsics ■ Sensation & reflexes WNL ■ (–) EMG; x-ray may show calcaneal spur but there is no correlation between a bone spur & pain of plantarfascitis
Tarsal Tunnel—compression of contents of tarsal tunnel (posterior tibial nerve & artery, tibialis posterior, FDL, FHL) may be 2° trauma, weight gain, excessive pronation, or inflammation	■ Sharp pain into medial/plantar aspect of foot & 1st MTP ■ Burning, nocturnal pain, swelling ■ ↑ Pain with walking & passive d-flexion or eversion ■ Motor weakness & intrinsic atrophy is difficult to detect ■ DTRs & ROM = WNL ■ (+) Tinel's sign just below & behind the medial malleolus ■ Abnormal EMG; r/o diabetic neuropathy & neuroma

Continued

Pathology/Mechanism	Signs/Symptoms
Peroneal Tendonitis—structurally 3 anatomic sites where tendon passes through tunnel/passage with acute angulation that can result in irritation & ↓ vascularization 2° trauma, inversion sprains, or direct blow	■ Subluxing tendon = snapping while everting in dorsiflexion; subluxation is more common in young athletes 2° to forceful dorsiflexion of inverted foot with peroneals contracting ■ Swelling & ecchymosis inferior to lateral malleolus ■ X-ray may show avulsion of peroneal retinaculum
Common Peroneal Nerve Palsy sitting with legs crossed, compression during sx, presence of a fabella (20% of population), tight ski boots or hockey skates, tx of nerve during strong inversion & plantarflexion contraction	■ Compromised ankle stability can ↑ risk of sprains ■ Local pain & ecchymosis at the site of external trauma ■ Foot drop, ↓ eversion & dorsiflexion ■ Partial sensory loss ■ Test = pain with walking on medial borders of foot ■ MRI, EMG/NCV may be helpful
Sever's Syndrome (Achilles Apophysitis)—occurs in 8–16 yo ♂>♀ 2° rapid growth with stress on epiphysis with jumping or athletic events; may occur (B)	■ Heel pain, TTP with mediolateral compression of calcaneus ■ ↓ Dorsiflexion due to pain; pain with stairs ■ Radiographs may not be helpful ■ Responds well to heel lift (healing takes months)
Achilles Tendonitis—vascular watershed is 4.5 cm above tendon insertion & vulnerable to ischemia 2° running hills (up = stretch & down = eccentric stress), poor footwear, excess pronation (↑ rotational forces); occurs mostly in ♂ 30–50 yo	■ Localized tenderness 2–6 cm proximal to Achilles insertion ■ Early morning stiffness, antalgic gait; pain climbing stairs ■ Tendon thickening & crepitus with AROM (wet leather) ■ Palpable Achilles nodule (retrocalcaneal exostosis = pump bump) ■ ↓ Ankle dorsiflexion with knee extended ■ MRI to r/o tendon defect & DVT

Continued

Pathology/Mechanism	Signs/Symptoms
Achilles Tendon Rupture—<30 yo, injury is 2° direct blow to gastroc or forceful contraction; >30 yo, injury is 2° degeneration (higher incidence in people with type "O" blood)	■ Snap/pop associated with injury ■ Palpable gap in tendon (hatchet sign) if examined early ■ Cannot walk on toes, swelling (within 1–2 hrs) & ecchymosis ■ (+) Thompson's test ■ MRI confirms diagnosis
Posterior Tibialis Tendonitis—inflammatory condition due to poor biomechanics or overuse; common in ♀ >40 yo	■ TTP @ medial ankle ■ Crepitus with AROM ■ Pain with passive pronation & active supination ■ Pain with resistive inversion & plantarflexion
Shin Splints/Anterior—an overuse syndrome of tibialis anterior, ext hallicus longus, & ext digitorum longus attributed to running on unconditioned legs, soft tissue imbalance, alignment abnormalities, & excessive pronation to accommodate rearfoot varus	■ Pain & tenderness over anterior tibialis ■ Pain with resisted dorsiflexion & inversion ■ Pain with stretching into plantarflexion & eversion ■ Callus formation under 2nd metatarsal head & medial side of distal hallux ■ Tight gastroc/soleus muscle ■ Soreness with heel walking ■ (−) X-ray, needed to r/o stress fx
Shin Splints/Posterior—an overuse syndrome of flexor hallucis longus & flexor digitorum longus	■ Callus formation under 2nd > 3rd > 4th MT head & medial side of distal hallux ■ Pain & soreness over distal 1/3–2/3 of posterior/medial shin & posterior medial malleolus ■ Hypermobile 1st metatarsal ■ Rapid & excessive pronation to compensate for rearfoot varus; result is ↑ stress on tibialis posterior to decelerate foot ■ Pain with resisted inversion & plantarflexion ■ Pain with stretching into dorsiflexion & eversion ■ (−) X-ray, needed to r/o stress fx

Continued

Pathology/Mechanism	Signs/Symptoms

Compartment Syndrome—a progression of shin splints resulting in a loss of microcirculation in shin muscle; ♂ > ♀, R > L
Beware: Immediate referral is needed (Ice but do not compress)
	■ 5 P's = paresthesia (toes), paresis (drop foot), pain (anterior tibia), pallor, pulseless
	■ Skin feels warm & firm
	■ Pain with stretch or AROM, foot drop
	■ Severe cramping, diffuse pain & tightness
	■ Most reliable sign is sensory deficit at the dorsum of foot in 1st interdigital cleft
	■ Ischemia of extensor hallicus longus
	■ Pulses are normal until the end & then surgery is needed within 4–6 hours is required to prevent muscle necrosis & nerve damage
	■ ↑ Soft tissue pressures via fluid accumulation
	  ■ Normal compartment pressure <10 mm Hg
	  ■ > 20 mm Hg is compromised capillary blood flow
	  ■ > 30 mm Hg results in ischemic necrosis
	■ (−) X-ray & bone scan; need to r/o tibial stress fx
	■ Confirmed with MRI & pressure assessment

Complex Regional Pain Syndrome—etiology unknown, may occur after trauma See stages on page 222.	■ Hyperalgesia & hyperhidrosis ■ Capsular tightness & stiffness ■ Muscle atrophy & osteoporosis ■ Trophic changes & edema ■ Vasomotor instability

Continued

Pathology/Mechanism	Signs/Symptoms
Syndesmotic Sprain—injury to anterior and/or posterior inferior tibiofibular ligament 2° hyperdorsiflexion & eversion See stages below	■ (+) Tests: Squeeze & ER test ■ Pain & swelling over ligament/ interosseous membrane ■ Oblique x-ray may show abnormal widening of joint space ■ Recovery time = 5 + (0.97 x cm from ankle joint that squeeze test is positive) ± 3 days ■ Need to r/o fx & avulsion
Lateral Sprain—injury to ATF, CF, PTF 2° inversion with plantarflexion See stages below	■ Rich blood supply = significant swelling within 2 hours ■ TTP over involved ligaments, ecchymosis that drains distal ■ Varying levels of instability (grade 1–3) ■ (+) Tests: Talar tilt & anterior drawer (presence of a dimple just inferior to the tip of the lateral malleolus) ■ (–) X-ray for fracture but stress film may show ↑ joint space ■ Arthrography is only accurate within 24 hours

Grades of Ankle Sprains

1st degree	2nd degree	3rd degree
■ No hemorrhage ■ Minimal swelling ■ Point tender ■ No varus laxity ■ (–)Anterior drawer ■ (–) Talar tilt ■ No/little limp ■ Difficulty hopping ■ Recovery 2–10 days	■ Some hemorrhage ■ Localized swelling (↓ Achilles definition) ■ (+) Anterior drawer ■ (+) Talar tilt ■ No varus laxity ■ (+) Limp ■ Unable to heel raise, hop, run ■ Recovery 10–30 days	■ Diffuse swelling (no Achilles definition) ■ Tenderness medial & lateral ■ (+) Anterior drawer ■ (+) Talar tilt ■ (+) Varus laxity ■ NWB ■ Recovery 30–90 days

References

Akseki D, Ozcan O, Boya H, Pinar H. A new weight-bearing meniscal test and a comparison with McMurray's test and joint line tenderness. *Arthroscopy*. 2004;20(9):951-958.

Albeck M. A critical assessment of clinical diagnosis of disc herniation in patients with monoradicular sciatica. *Acta Neurochiropractic*. 1996;138:40-44.

Albert H, Godskesen M, Westergaard J. Evaluation of clinical tests used in classification procedures in pregnancy-related pelvic joint pain. *European Spine Journal*. 2000;9(2):161-166.

Arky R (Medical Consultant). *Physicians' Desk Reference*. Montvocle, NJ: Medical Economics Company. 2008

Barankin B, Freiman A. *Derm Notes*. Philadelphia, PA: FA Davis; 2006.

Barth JRH, Burkhart SS, DeBeer JF. Bear-Hug Test: A New and Sensitive Test for Diagnosing a Subscapular Tear. *Arthroscopy: The Journal of Arthroscopy and Related Surgery*. October 2006;22(10):1076-1084.

Beaton DE, Wright JG, Katz JN. Development of the Quick DASH: Comparison of three item-reduction approaches. *The Journal of Bone and Joint Surgery*. May 2005;87A(5):1038-1046.

Bellamy N, Buchanan WW, et al. Validation study of WOMAC: A health status instrument for measuring clinically important patient relevant outcomes to antirheumatic drug therapy in patients with osteoarthritis of the hip or knee. *Journal of Rheumatology*. 1988;15:1833-1840.

Bellamy N. Pain assessment in osteoarthritis: Experience with the WOMAC osteoarthritis index. *Seminars in Arthritis and Rheumatism*. 1989;18 (supplement 2):14-17.

Benner W. Specificity of the Speed's test: Arthroscopic technique for evaluating the biceps tendon at the level of the bicipital groove. *Arthroplasty*. 1998;14(8):789-796.

Biel A. *Trail Guide to the Body*. 2nd ed. Boulder, CO: Discovery Books; 2001.

Blower PW, Griffin AJ. Clinical sacroiliac tests in ankylosing spondylitis and other causes of low back pain. *Annals of Rheumatic Disorders*. 1984;43:192-195.

Boeree NR, Ackroyd CE. Assessment of the meniscus and cruciate ligaments: an audit of clinical practice. *Injury*. 1991;22(4):291-294.

Boissannault WG. *Primary Care for the Physical Therapist*. Elsevier Saunders, 2005

Boissannault WG, Bass C. Pathological origins of trunk and neck pain: Part I–Pelvic and abdominal visceral disorders. *Journal of Orthopedics and Sports Physical Therapy*. 1990;12(5):192-207.

Boissannault WG, Bass C. Pathological origins of trunk and neck pain: Part II–Disorders of the cardiovascular and pulmonary systems. *Journal of Orthopedics and Sports Physical Therapy*. 1990;12(5):208-215.

Boissannault WG, Bass C. Pathological origins of trunk and neck pain: Part III–Diseases of the musculoskeletal system. *Journal of Orthopedics and Sports Physical Therapy*. 1990;12(5):216-221.

Brantigan CO, Roos DB. Diagnosing thoracic outlet syndrome. *Hand Clinics*. 2004;20:27-36.

Broadhurst NA, Bond MJ. Pain provocation tests for the assessment of sacroiliac joint dysfunction. *Journal of Spinal Disorders*. 1998;11(4): 341-345.

Broomhead A, Stuart P. Validation of the Ottawa ankle rules in Australia. *Emergency Medicine*. 2003;15(2):126-132.

Bruske J, Bednarski M, Grzelec H, Zyluk A. The usefulness of the Phalen test and the Hoffman-Tinel sign in the diagnosis of carpal tunnel syndrome. *Acta Orthopaedica Belgica*. 2002;68(2):141-145.

Budiman-Mak E, Conrad KJ, Roach KF. The Foot Function Index: a measure of foot pain and disability. *Journal of Clinical Epidemiology*. 1991;44(6):561-570.

Burkhart S, Morgan CB, Kibler B. Shoulder injuries in overhead athletes: the dead arm revisited. *Clinics in Sports Medicine*. 2000;19(1):125-158.

Butler DA. *Mobilisation of the Nervous System*. Melbourne, Australia: Churchill Livingstone; 1991.

Cailliet R. *Hand Pain and Impairment*. 2nd ed. Philadelphia, PA: FA Davis; 1976.

Cailliet R. *Neck and Arm Pain*. Philadelphia, PA: FA Davis; 1976.

Cailliet R. *Foot and Ankle Pain*. Philadelphia, PA: FA Davis; 1976.

Cailliet R. *Knee Pain and Disability*. Philadelphia, PA: FA Davis; 1976.

Cailliet R. *Low Back Pain Syndrome*. 3rd ed. Philadelphia, PA: FA Davis; 1983.

Calis M, Akgen K, Birtane M, Calis H, Tuzun F. Diagnostic values of clinical diagnostic tests in subacromial impingement syndrome. *Annals of the Rheumatic Disease*. 2000;59:44-47.

Cibulka MT, Koldehoff R. Clinical usefulness of a cluster of sacroiliac joint tests in patients with and without low back pain. *Journal of Orthopedic and Sports Physical Therapy*. 1999;29(2):83-92.

Ciccone, CD. *Pharmacology in Rehabilitation*. 2nd ed. Philadelphia, PA: FA Davis; 1990.

Clark KD, Tanner S. Evaluation of the Ottawa ankle rules in children. *Pediatric Emergency Care*. 2003;19(2):73-78.

Colachis S, Ctrohm M. A study of tractive forces and angle of pull on vertebral interspaces in cervical spine. *Archives of Physical Medicine*. 1965;46:820-830.

Crocket HC, Gross LB, Wilk KE, Schwartz ML, Reed J, O'Mara J, Reilly MT, Dugas JR, Meister K, Lynam S, Andrews JR. Osseous adaptations and range of motion at the glenohumeral joint in professional baseball pitchers. *American Journal of Sports Medicine*. 2002; 30:20-26.

DeGarceau D, Dean D, Requejo SM, Thordarson DB. The association between diagnosis of plantar fasciitis and windlass test results. *Foot and Ankle International*. March 2003;24(3):251-255.

Deglin JH, Vallerand AH. *Davis's Drug Guide for Nurse*. 7th ed. Philadelphia, PA: FA Davis; 2001.

Duruoz MT, Poiraudeau S, Fermanian J, Menkes CJ, Amor B, Dougados M, Revel M. Development and validation of a rheumatoid hand functional disability scale that assesses functional handicap. *Journal of Rheumatology*. 1996; Jul;23(7):1167-1172.

Dutton M. *Orthopaedic Examination, Evaluation, and Intervention*. New York: McGraw Hill; 2004.

Dworkin SF, Huggins KH, LeResche L, Von Korff M, Howard J, Truelove E, Sommers E. Epidemiology of signs and symptoms in temporomandibular disorders: clinical signs in cases and controls. *Journal of the American Dental Association*. 1990;120(3):273-281.

Evans PJ, Bell GD, Frank C. Prospective evaluation of the McMurray test. *American Journal of Sports Medicine*. 1993;21(4):604-608.

Evans PJ. Prospective evaluation of the McMurray test. *American Journal of Sports Medicine*. 1994;22:567-568.

Evans R. *Illustrated Orthopedic Physical Assessment*. 2nd ed. St. Louis, MO: Mosby; 2001.

Fairbank JC, Couper J, Davies JB, O'Brien JP. The Oswestry low back pain disability questionnaire. *Physiotherapy*. 1980;66:271-273.

Farrell K. APTA Home Study Course, Solutions to Shoulder Disorders, 11.1.6 Adhesive Capsulitis.

Faught BE. Efficacy of clinical tests in the diagnosis of carpal tunnel. Doctoral dissertation, 2001.

Fitzgerald RH Jr. Acetabular labrum tears: diagnosis and treatment. *Clinical Orthopedics*. 1995;311:60-68.

Fowler PJ, Lubliner JA. The predictive value of five clinical signs in the evaluation of meniscal pathology. *Arthroscopy*. 1989;5:184-186.

Gann N. *Orthopedics at a Glance*. Thorofare, NJ: Slack Incorporated; 2001.

Gillard J, Perez-Cousin M, Hachulla E, Remy J, Hurtevent J-F, Vinckier L, Thevenon A, Duquesnoy B. Ddiagnosing thoracic outlet syndrome: contribution of provocative tests, ultrasonography, electrophysiology, and helical computer tomography In 48 patients. *Joint Bone Spine.* 2001;68416-424.

Goloborod'ko SA. Provocative test for carpal tunnel syndrome. *Journal of Hand Therapy.* 2004;17:344-348.

Goodman C, Boissonnault W. *Pathology: Implications for the Physical Therapist.* Philadelphia, PA: W.B. Saunders; 1998.

Goodman C, Snyder T. *Differential Diagnosis for Physical Therapists: Screening for Referral.* 4th ed. Philadelphia, PA: W.B. Saunders; 2008.

Guanche CA, Jones DC. Clinical testing for tears of the glenoid labrum. *Arthroscopy.* 2003;19(5):517-523.

Gulick DT. *Sport Notes.* Philadelphia, PA: FA Davis, 2008.

Gulick DT. *Screening Notes.* Philadelphia, PA: FA Davis, 2006

Hall CM, Brody LT. *Therapeutic Exercise.* Philadelphia, PA: Lippincott Williams and Wilkins; 1998.

Hall H. A simple approach to back pain management. *Patient Care.* 1992;15: 77-91.

Hansen PA, Micklesen P, Robinson LR. Clinical utility of the flick maneuver in diagnosing carpal tunnel syndrome. *American Journal of Physical Medicine and Rehabilitation.* 2004;83:363-367.

Harilainen A. Evaluation of knee instability in acute ligamentous injuries. *Annal of Chiropractic Gynaecology.* 1987;76:269-273.

Harris H. Harris hip score. *Journal of Bone and Joint Surgery (Am).* 1969;51-A(4):737-55.

Heald SL, Riddle DL, Lamb RL. The shoulder pain and disability index: The construct validity and responsiveness of a region-specific disability measure. *Physical Therapy,* 1997;77:1079-1089.

Hegedus EJ, Goode A, Campbell S, Morin A, Tamaddoni M, Moorman CT, Cook C. Physical examination of the shoulder: a systematic review with meta-analysis of the individual tests. *British Journal of Sports Medicine.* 2008;42:80-92.

Heller L, Ring H, Costeff H, Solzi P. Evaluation of Tinel's and Phalen's signs in diagnosis of the carpal tunnel syndrome. *European Neurology.* 1986;25(1):40-42.

Hertel R, Ballmer FT, Lambert SM, Gerber CH. Lag signs in the diagnosis of rotator cuff rupture. *Journal of Shoulder and Elbow Surgery.* 1996;5(4):307-313.

Holtby MB, et al. Accuracy of the Speed's and Yergason tests in detecting biceps pathology and slap lesions: comparison with arthroscopic findings. *Arthroscopy.* 2004;20(3):231-236.

Holtby MB, Razmjou H. Validity of the supraspinatus test as a single clinical test in diagnosing patients with rotator cuff pathology. *Journal of Orthopedics and Sports Physical Therapy.* 2004;34:194-200.

Hoppenfeld S. *Physical Examination of the Spine and Extremities.* New York, NY: Appleton-Century-Crofts; 1976.

Institute for Work and Health. http://www.iwh.on.ca/products/dash.php. Accessed February 2008.

Internet Drug Index. Available at: http://www.rxlist.com. Accessed August 2004.

Johanson M. APTA Home Study Course, Solutions to Shoulder Disorders, 11.1.4 Rotator Cuff Disorders.

Itoi E, Kido T, Sano A, Urayama M, Sata K. Which is more useful, the "full can test" or the "empty can test" in detecting the torn supraspinatus tendon? *American Journal of Sports Medicine.* 1999;27:65-68.

Jonsson T, Althoff B, Peterson L, Renstrom P. Clinical diagnosis of ruptures of the anterior cruciate ligament: a comparative study of the Lachman test and the anterior drawer sign. *American Journal of Sports Medicine.* 1982;10:100-102.

Kaikkonen A, Kannus P, Jarvinen M. A performance test protocol and scoring scale for the evaluation of ankle injuries. *American Journal of Sports Medicine.* 1994;22(4):462-469.

Karachalios T, Hantes M, Zibis AH, Zachos V, Karantanas AH, Malizos KN. Diagnostic accuracy of a new clinical test (the Thessaly test) for early detection of meniscal tears. *Journal of Bone and Joint Surgery.* May 2005; 87A(5):955-962.

Katz JW, Fingeroth RJ. The diagnostic accuracy of ruptures of the anterior cruciate ligament comparing the Lachman test, the anterior drawer sign, and the pivot shift test in acute and chronic knee injuries. *American Journal of Sports Medicine.* 1986;14(1):88-91.

Khine H, Dorfman DH, Avner JR. Applicability of Ottawa knee rules for knee injuries in children. *Pediatric Emergency Care.* 2001;17(6):401-404.

Kim S-H, Ha, K-I, Ahn J-H, Kim S-H, Choi H-J. Biceps load test II: a clinical test for SLAP lesions of the shoulder. *Arthroscopy.* 2001;17(2):160-164.

Kim S-H, Park J-S, Jeong W-K, Shin S-K. The Kim test. *American Journal of Sports Medicine.* 2005;33(8):1188-1192.

Knuttson B. Comparative value of electromyographic, and clinical-neurological examinations in diagnosis of lumbar root compression syndrome. *Acta Orthopedic Scandinavia.* 1961;Suppl 49:19-49.

Kosteljanetz M, Espersen O, Halaburt H, Miletic T. Predictive values of clinical and surgical findings in patients with lumbago-sciatica: a prospective study. *Acta Neurochirugica.* 1984;73:67-76.

Kuhlman KA, Hennessey WJ. Sensitivity and specificity of carpal tunnel syndrome signs. *American Journal of Physical Medicine and Rehabilitation.* 1997;76(6):451-457.

Kurosaka M, Yagi M, Yoshiya S, Muratsu H, Mizuno K. Efficiency of the axially loaded pivot shift test for the diagnosis of a meniscal tear. *International Orthopedics*. 1999;23:271-274.

Lan LB. The scaphoid shift test. *The Journal of Hand Surgery*. 1993;18A(2): 366-368.

Laslett M, Aprill CN, McDonald B, Young SB. Diagnosis of sacroiliac joint pain: validity of individual provocation tests and composites of tests. *Manual Therapy*. 2005;10:207-218.

Laslett M, Young SB, Aprill CN, McDonald B. Diagnosing painful sacroiliac joints: a validity study of a McKenzie evaluation and sacroiliac provocation tests. *Australian Journal of Physiotherapy*. 2003;49:89-97.

LaStayo P, Weiss S. The GRIT: a quantitative measure of ulnar impaction syndrome. *Journal of Hand Therapy*. 2001;14(3):173-179.

Lee JK, Yao L, Phelps CT, Wirth CR, Czajka J, Lozman J. Anterior cruciate ligament tears: MR imaging compared with arthroscopy and clinical tests. *Radiology*. 1988;166:861-864.

Leroux, et al. Diagnostic value of clinical tests for shoulder impingement syndrome. *Revue du Rhumatisme*. 1995;62(6):423-428.

Lester B, Halbrecht J, Levy IM, Gaudinez R. "Press test" for office diagnosis of triangular fibrocartilage complex tears of the wrist. *Annals of Plastic Surgery*. 1995;35(1):41-45.

Levangie PK. Four clinical tests of sacroiliac joint dysfunction: the association of test results with innominate torsion among patients with and without low back pain. *Physical Therapy*. 1999;79(11):1043-1057.

Levangie PK, Norkin CC. *Joint Structure and Function*. 3rd ed. Philadelphia, PA: FA Davis; 2001.

Levine DW, Simmons BP, Koris MJ, Daltroy LH, Hohl GG, Fossel AH, Katz JN. A self-administered questionnaire for the assessment of severity of symptoms and functional status in carpal tunnel syndrome. *Journal of Bone and Joint Surgery*. 1993;75(11):1585-1592.

Lewis C, McNerney T. *Clinical Measures of Functional Outcomes*. Virginia: Learn Publications.

Lewis CL, Sahrmann SA. Acetabular labral tears. *Physical Therapy*. 2006; 86(1):110-121.

Lewis CL, Sahrmann SA, Moran DW. Anterior hip joint force increases with hip extension, decreased gluteal force, or decreased iliopsoas force. *Journal of Biomechanics*. 2007;40:3725-3731.

Lewis C, Wilk K, Wright R. *The Orthopedic OutcomesTool Box*. Virginia: Learn Publications.

Lillegard WA, Burcher JD, Rucker KS. *Handbook of Sports Medicine*. 2nd ed. Boston, MA: Butterworth-Heinemann; 1999.

Liu SH, Henry MH, Nuccion SL. A prospective evaluation of a new physical examination in predicting glenoid labral tears. *American Journal of Sports Medicine.* 1996;24(6):721-725.

Liu SH, Osti L, Henry M, Bocchi L. The diagnosis of acute complete tears of the anterior cruciate ligament. Comparison of MRI, arthrometry and clinical examination. *Journal of Bone and Joint Surgery.* 1995;77(4): 586-588.

Lo IKY, Nonweiler B, Woolfrey M, Litchfield R, Kirkley A. An evaluation of the apprehension, relocation, and surprise tests for anterior shoulder instability. *American Journal of Sports Medicine.* 2004;32(3):655-661.

Lucchesi GM, Jackson RE, Peacock WF, Cerasani C, Swor RA. Sensitivity of the Ottawa rules. *Annals of Emergency Medicine.* 1995;26(1);1-5.

Ludewig P. APTA Home Study Course, Solutions to Shoulder Disorders, 11.1.1 Functional Shoulder Anatomy and Biomechanics.

Lysholm J, Gillquist J. Evaluation of knee ligament surgery results with special emphasis on using of a scoring scale. *American Journal of Sports Medicine.* 1982;10:150-154.

MacDermid JC, Turgeon T, Richards RS, Beadle M, Roth JH. Patient rating of wrist pain and disability: a reliable and valid measurement tool. *Journal of Orthopaedic Trauma.* November 1998;12(8):577-586.

MacDermid JC, Wessel J. Clinical diagnosis of carpal tunnel syndrome: a systemic review. *Journal of Hand Therapy.* 2004;17(2):309-319.

MacDonald PB, Clark P, Sutherland K. An analysis of the diagnostic accuracy of the Hawkins and Neer subacromial impingement tests. *Journal of Shoulder and Elbow Surgery.* 2000;9(4):299-301.

Magee D. *Orthopedic Physical Assessment.* 4th ed. Philadelphia: WB Saunders; 2002.

Malanga GA, Andrus S, Nadler SF, McLean J. Physical examination of the knee: a review of the original test description and scientific validity of common orthopedic tests. *Archives of Physical Medicine and Rehabilitation.* 2003;84:592-603.

Martin RL, Sekiya JK. The interrater reliability of 4 clinical tests used to assess individuals with musculoskeletal hip pain. *Journal of Orthopedics and Sports Physical Therapy.* 2008;38(2):71-77

McFarland EG, Kim TK, Savino RM. Clinical assessment of three common tests for superior labral anterior-posterior lesions. *American Journal of Sports Medicine.* 2002;30(6):810-815.

McKinnis LN. *Fundamentals of Orthopedic Radiology.* Philadelphia, PA: FA Davis; 1997.

Medscape from Web MD. Available at: www.medscape.com. Accessed August 2004.

Melzack R. The McGill pain questionnaire. In: *Pain Measurement and Assessment*. New York: Raven Press; 1983:41-48.

Melzack R. The short-form McGill pain questionnaire. *Pain*. 1987;30:191-197.

Mimori K, Muneta T, Nakagawa T, Shinomiya K. A new pain provocation test for superior labral tears of the shoulder. *American Journal of Sports Medicine*. 1999;27:137-142.

Nakagawa S, Yoneda M, Hayashida K, Obata M, Fukushima S, Miyazaki Y. Forced shoulder abduction and elbow flexion test: a new simple clinical test to detect superior labral injury in the throwing shoulder. *Arthroscopy*. 2005;21(11):1290-1295.

Narvani A, Tsiridis E, Kendall S, Chaudhuri R, Thomas P. A preliminary report on prevalence of acetabular labrum tears in sport patients with groin pain. *Knee Surgery, Traumatology, and Arthroscopy*. 2003;11:403-408.

Neumann D. *Kinesiology of the Musculoskeletal System*. St. Louis, MO: Mosby; 2002.

Nils J, van Geel C, van der Auwera, van de Velde B. Diagnostic value of five clinical tests in patellofemoral pain syndrome. *Manual Therapy*. 2005

Noble J, Erat K. In defense of the meniscus: a prospective study of 200 meniscectomy patients. *Journal of Bone and Joint Surgery*. 1980;62-B:7–11.

Novak CB, Lee GW, Mackinnon SE, Lay L. Provocation testing for cubital tunnel syndrome. Journal of Hand Surgery. 1994;19A:817-820.

O'Brien SJ, Pagnani MJ, Fealy S, McGlynn SR, Wilson JB. The active compression test: A new and effective test for diagnosing labral tears and acromioclavicular joint abnormality. American Journal of Sports Medicine. 1998;26(5):610-613.

Park HB, Yokota A, Gill HS, Rassi GE, McFarland EG. Diagnostic accuracy of clinical tests for the different degrees of subacromial impingement syndrome. Journal of Bone and Joint Surgery. 2005;87-A(7):1446-1455.

Partentis MA, Mohr KJ, ElAttrache NS. Disorders of the superior labrum: review and treatment guidelines. *Clinical Orthopedics*. 2002;400:77-87.

Pfalzer LA, Drouin J. Screening for underlying cancer in acute care physical therapy practice. *Acute Care Perscpectives*. 2001;10(1-2):1-4,10,14,17,36, 40,44-55.

Flint AC, Bulloch D, Osmand MU, Stiell L, Dunlap H, Reed M, Tenenhein M, Klassen TP. Validation of the Ottawa ankle rules in children with ankle injuries. *Academic Emergency Medicine*. 1999;6(10):1005-1009.

Powell JM, Lloyd GJ, Rintoul RF. New clinical test for fracture of the scaphoid. *Canadian Journal of Surgery*. July 1988;31(4):237-242.

Ransford AO, Cairns D, Mooney V. The pain drawing as an aid to the psychoReider B. *The Orthopedic Physical Examination*. Philadelphia, PA: WB Saunders Company; 1999.

Rayan GM, Jensen C. Thoracic outlet syndrome: provocative examination maneuvers in a typical population. *Journal of Shoulder and Elbow Surgery*. 1995;4:113-117.

Roach KE. Development of a shoulder pain and disability index. Arthritis Care and Research. *1991;4:*143-149.

Rothstein JM, Roy SH, Wolf SL. *The Rehabilitation Specialist's Handbook*. Philadelphia, PA: FA Davis; 1991.

Rubinstein RA Jr, Shelbourne KD, McCarroll JR, VanMeter CD, Rettig AC. The accuracy of the clinical examination in the setting of posterior cruciate ligament injuries. *American Journal of Sports Medicine*. 1994;22:550-557.

Russell A, Maksymovich W, LeClerq S. Clinical examination of the sacroiliac joints. A prospective study. *Arthritis and Rheumatism*. 1981;24:1575-1577.

Saal JA. Natural history and nonoperative treatment of lumbar disk herniation. *Spine*. 1996;21(24S):7S.

Saidoff D, McDonough A. *Critical Pathways in Therapeutic Intervention*. St. Louis, MO, Mosby; 2002.

Sallay PI, Poggi J, Speer KP, Garrett WE. Acute dislocation of the patella. A correlation pathoanatomic study. *American Journal of Sports Medicine*. 1996;24:52-60.

Sandberg R, Balkfors B, Henricson A, Westlin N. Stability tests in knee ligament injuries. *Archives of Orthopedic Trauma Surgery*. 1986;106(1):5-7.

Saunders HD, Ryan RS. *Evaluation, Treatment and Prevention of Musculoskeletal Disorders*. Volume 1-Spine. 4th ed. Chaska, MN: The Saunders Group; 2004.

Scalzitti DA. Screening for psychological factors in patients with low back problems: Waddell's nonorganic signs. *Physical Therapy*. 1997; 77 (3):306-312.

Scholten RJPM, Deville WLJM, Opstelten W, Bijl D, Van der Plas CG, Bouter LM. The accuracy of physical diagnostic tests for assessing meniscal lesions of the knee. *Journal of Family Practice*. 2001;50(11):938-944.

Sgaglione NA, Pizzo WD, Fox JM, Friedman MJ. Critical analysis of knee ligament rating systems. *American Journal of Sports Medicine*. 1995;23(6): 660-667.

Stankovic R, Johnell O, Maly P, Willner S. Use of lumbar extension, slump test, physical and neurological examination in the evaluation of patients with suspected herniated nucleus pulposus. A prospective clinical study. *Manual Therapy*. 1999;4(1):25-32.

Starkey C, Ryan J. *Orthopedic and Athletic Injury Evaluation Handbook*. Philadelphia, PA: FA Davis; 2003.

Stiell IG, McKnight RD, Greenberg GH, McDowell I, Nair RC, Wells GA, Johns C, Worthington JR. Implementation of the Ottawa ankle rules. *JAMA*. March 1994;271(11):827-832.

Stiell IG, Wells GA, Hoag RH. Implementation of the Ottawa knee rule for the use of radiography in acute knee injuries. *JAMA*, 1997;278:2075-2079.

Stiell IG, Greenberg GH, Well GA, McDowell I, Cwinn AA, Smith NA et al. Prospective validation of a decision rule for the use of radiography in acute knee injuries. JAMA. 1996,275:611-615.

Stratford PW, Binkley J. A review of the McMurray test: definition, interpretation, and clinical usefulness. *Journal of Orthopedic and Sports Physical Therapy*. 1995;22(3):116-120.

Suenaga E, Noguchi Y, Jingushi S, Shuto T, Nakashima Y, Miyanishi K, Iwamoto Y. Relationship between the maximum flexion-internal rotation test and the torn acetabular labrum of a dysplastic hip. *Journal of Orthopedic Science*. 2002;7:26-32.

Szabo RM, Slater RR. Diagnostic testing in carpal tunnel syndrome. *Journal of Hand Surgery*. 2000;25(1):184.

Tegner Y, Lysholm J. Rating system in the evaluation of knee ligament injuries. *Clinical Orthopedics*. 1985;198:43-49.

Tennet DT, Beach WR, Meyers JF. Clinical sports medicine update. A review of the special tests associated with shoulder examination. *American Journal of Sports Medicine*. 2003;31:154-160.

Tetro AM, Evanoff BA, Hollstien SB, Gelberman RH. A new provocation test for carpal tunnel syndrome. Assessment of wrist flexion and nerve compression. *Journal of Bone and Joint Surgery*. 1998;80(3):493-498.

Thompson JC. *Netter's Concise Atlas of Orthopedic Anatomy*. Teterboro, NJ: Icon Learning Systems; 2002.

Tigges S, Pitts S, Mukundan S Jr, Morrison D, Olson M, Shahriara A. External validation of the Ottawa knee rules in an urban trauma center in the United States. *American Journal of Roentgenology*. 1999;172(4):1069-1071.

Tomberlin J. APTA Home Study Course, Solutions to Shoulder Disorders, 11.1.2 Physical Diagnostic Tests of the Shoulder: An Evidence-based Perspective.

Tong HC, Haig AJ, Yamakawa K. Spurling test and cervical radiculopathy. *Spine*. 2002;27(2):156-159.

Torg JS, Conrad W, Kalen V. Clinical diagnosis of anterior cruciate ligament instability in the athlete. *American Journal of Sports Medicine*. 1976;4: 84-93.

Travell J, Simon D. *Trigger Point Flip Charts*. Baltimore, MD: Williams and Wilkins; 1996.

Unverzagt CA, Schuemann T, Mathisen J. Differential diagnosis of a sports hernia in a high-school athlete. *Journal of Orthopedics and Sports Physical Therapy*. 2008;38(2):63-70.

Ure BM, Tiling T, Kirchner R, Rixen D. Reliability of clinical examination of the shoulder in comparison with arthroscopy. *Unfallchirurg*. 1993;96: 382-386.

Van der Wurff P, Meyne W, Hagmeijer RHM. Clinical tests of the sacroiliac joint. *Manual Therapy*. 2000;5(2):89-96.

Vernon H, Mior S. The Neck Disability Index: A study of reliability and validity. *Journal of Manipulative and Physiological Therapeutics*. 1991;14:409-415.

Waddell G. Nonorganic physical signs in low back pain. *Spine*. 1980; 5(2): 117-125.

Waddell G, McCulloch JA, Kummel E, Venner RM. Nonorganic physical signs in low-back pain. *Spine*. 1980; 5:117-125.

Wainner RS, Fritz JM, Irrgang JJ, Boninger ML, Delitto A, Allison S. Reliability and diagnostic accuracy of the clinical examination and patient self-report measures for cervical radiculopathy. *Spine*. 2003;28(1):52-62.

Wainner RS, Boninger ML, Balu G, Burdett R, Helkowski W. Durkan gauge and carpal compression test: accuracy and diagnostic test properties. *Journal of Orthopedic and Sports Physical Therapy*. 2000;30(11):676-682.

Wolf EM, Agrawal V. Transdeltoid palpation (the rent sign) in the diagnosis of rotator cuff tears. *Journal of Shoulder and Elbow Surgery*. 2001;10(5):470-473.

For an expanded index go to, http://davisplus.fadavis.com, Keyword, Gulick

For an expanded index go to, http://davisplus.fadavis.com, Keyword, Gulick

For an expanded index go to, http://davisplus.fadavis.com, Keyword, Gulick

For an expanded index go to, http://davisplus.fadavis.com, Keyword, Gulick

For an expanded index go to, http://davisplus.fadavis.com, Keyword, Gulick